GUARDED PROGNOSIS

A Doctor and His Patients Talk about

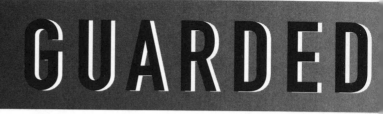

GUARDED

Chronic Disease and How to Cope with It

PROGNOSIS

MICHAEL LOCKSHIN, M.D.

HILL AND WANG

A DIVISION OF FARRAR, STRAUS AND GIROUX / NEW YORK

Hill and Wang
A division of Farrar, Straus and Giroux
19 Union Square West, New York 10003

Library of Congress Cataloging-in-Publication Data
Lockshin, Michael D., 1937–
    Guarded prognosis / Michael D. Lockshin.
        p.   cm.
    Includes index.
    ISBN 0-8090-5345-4
    1. Musculoskeletal system—Diseases—Case studies.   2. Systemic
lupus erythematosus—Case studies.   3. Lockshin, Michael D., 1937–.
5. Medical care—United States.   6. Medicaid.   7. Medicare.
I. Title.
RC925.5.L63   1998
362.1'0973—dc21   98-10735

TO JANE

for a lifetime of inspiration

CONTENTS

ACKNOWLEDGMENTS

I am grateful to my patients, both the few described in these pages and many others, for sharing their personal thoughts and for allowing me to learn from them.

As this book evolved, people close to me tolerated incessant conversations about it and read many versions of it. In particular, I thank my father and mother. I am glad that they lived long enough to read and offer suggestions for the first two drafts. My wife, Jane, and my daughter, Amanda, were my severest and most thoughtful critics; they dissected illogical and often ambiguous grammar with intensity, but not malice, and compulsively questioned the accuracy of some of my facts. Any errors that remain are my own fault. Other Lockshins were also very helpful in their comments—Richard and Zahra, Miriam, Nora, Sheila and Norman—as was my brother-in-law, Alan Roberts. Isadore Rosenfeld critiqued my first draft, then walked me through the steps of how a book is published. Robert and Julie Bailey, Lawrence Small, Lewis and Janet Solomon, and Susan Dollinger, and Allen Ermann added economic and other insights. Ellen and Bud Gibbs, and Alida Brill challenged me with insightful conversation.

Alan Kellock, my agent, understood my intent; I am grateful for his enthusiastic support. Elisabeth Sifton, in editing, showed me structure and organization, and helped me turn the draft into a finished book.

GUARDED PROGNOSIS

INTRODUCTION

If I do not speak for myself, who will be for me?
And being for myself, what am I?
And if not now, when?
—PIRKE ABOTH (*ETHICS OF THE FATHERS*)

In my real world at work, I wear a long white coat. A stethoscope bounces in the pocket as I walk, its weight a comfort to me. The coat is made of a synthetic fabric, and its pockets are loose, so the earpieces of the stethoscope fly free when my gait is brisk. In the hospital, at the nurses' station, I pause to write down formal medical details in my patients' charts.

At other times, my white coat is off and I transcribe a larger, more informal tale. I say "transcribe," because the stories I have written down here have been dictated by the actions of my patients and other people who determine the fates of the chronically ill.

This is a book of stories about real Americans, about their medical problems, and about the effects on their lives of changing medical-care policies. Parallel to each patient's medical problem is a social problem. These problems contrast and sometimes conflict with what may be best for the nation as a whole. As a doctor, I have seen that when the policies change, the personal stories also change. In each of the stories I tell here, different values are juxtaposed—those of the individual and those of society. Each story asks: What happens to those for whom the medical safety net is only a sometime thing?

For thirty-five years I have observed the effect of changing medical-care policy on my patients. Then, working in the government, I learned what should have been but was not obvious to me: that policy comes from public will, and there is no good policy without knowledge. The best way to promote knowledge is through examples. Stories about people are more accessible than statistical analysis.

These are stories about people whose medical support is or was at risk when policies changed.* I hope the reader will con-

---

*Many of the patients I describe have a disease that doctors call lupus, or SLE, short for its mouth-filling full name, systemic lupus erythematosus. A word about what lupus is will therefore be useful. (Other patients in this book have more familiar diagnoses, rheumatoid arthritis and osteoarthritis, and still others have rare diagnoses, scleroderma and Takayasu's arteritis.)

No one knows the cause of lupus. What is known is that lupus primarily attacks young women, particularly young women of color, and that it can be quite mild or very dangerous. (Most patients with lupus are less sick than are the patients described in these pages.) Lupus causes rashes, arthritis, kidney failure, and a variety of brain problems.

Because of fear that the disease would worsen, until the 1980s women with lupus were told never to become pregnant. I was fortunate to be practicing when lupus patients, then their doctors, discovered they could safely carry children. Pregnancy, with all its ethical and fiscal implications, appears frequently in these stories.

Lupus is a good focal point for a study of a health-care system because it affects every organ in the body and because it comes and goes in cycles over long periods of time. Lupus patients use all segments of the medical-care system, including research. Patients with lupus may need our most exotic technology; being mostly young, they have marvelous powers of recovery, which makes extending maximal medical effort always appropriate.

sider deeply, and with feeling, the personal consequences of those changes. I want this to happen because I believe that those who are ill—particularly those with chronic illness, those who are poor, and those who cannot speak for themselves— have not been heard in the debate about medical care in America today. The ill need advocates. Not all can speak for themselves. If their doctors do not speak for them, who will?

I hope these tales prompt the reader to think about the tension that exists between individual and public values in health matters, to think about how we decide what we must do. Do we choose differently when individuals are the focus of our concern? When entire populations are?

My stories are about patients I have treated. I have drawn heavily on my experience as a physician—or, rather, on the experiences of patients who have come under my care. Each story is true, though names and identifying details have of course been changed.*

The stories begin more than three decades ago. Access to medical care in the early 1960s was a chancy thing. In that era, when access was denied, it was a passive denial, not an active one. The criterion was personal wealth, and hospital doors were open if the patient could pay. From the late 1960s, after Medicare and Medicaid, that chanciness nearly vanished. Universal access was the norm, and it remains so until this day. But now, at the end of the century, we are about to em-

---

They touch, and put stress on, almost every aspect of the health-care system.

*When I make someone's cultural or racial background obvious, it is because the person made it clear to me that this was important. Political correctness is an appropriate goal for policy, but ignoring the ethnic or economic or racial background makes for bad doctoring. In any case, political correctness does not make ethnicity disappear, and so I have not tried to hide ethnicity here.

bark on an ugly journey to a land where patients' access to
care is actively denied, where patients are refused care if the
public or the corporation, not the individual, is unable or unwilling to pay. Those who would pay the bill look into their
wallets and prejudge: Your illness will be expensive; to care for
you will be costly; you may not enter here. Human kindness
is for sale. It need not be this way.

There are other choices. To raise the questions, to initiate
a debate, to amplify the voices of those who need to be heard,
this book asks: How much does compassion cost? Should
"health" care be given only to the healthy—no ill need apply?

Who elected those whose job is to be inhumane? By what
authority do they rule?

BELLEVUE AND SMALL-TOWN MEDICINE

In the spring of 1961, before there was Medicare, Dr. David
Rutstein challenged a second-year medical-school class with an
assignment. He described four patients; the assignment was
for us students to use our spring recess to learn how each of
these patients would be cared for in a given place—our home-
towns, or anywhere we chose. One had chronic mental illness,
another had tuberculosis, another needed extensive surgery,
and the fourth was (I think—it's been a long time) a mal-
nourished child. The point was, none of these four patients
could afford medical care. (I later understood that the assignment had had a basic flaw: we students were sent to interview
doctors, but we did not talk to patients.)

To write my answer, I visited a very small town in which
my uncle was a general practitioner, the type of GP whose
patients often paid in chickens and eggs instead of cash. I
learned that, in Mount Vernon, Ohio, charity, state hospitals,

and luck kept the wolves from people's doors. Yet my uncle was certain that none of the four would lack medical care. Dr. Rutstein's lesson has stayed with me for thirty-five years.

Two and a half years later I had finished medical school. I was a medical resident at Bellevue, the great charity hospital in lower Manhattan. It was at Bellevue that I began to see the patients' side of the story.

Bellevue was an imposing Victorian anachronism, a sooty red-brick building with gray concrete cornices, all of it blackened with urban grime from time immemorial. Bellevue, perhaps once appropriately named, now overlooked Con Edison smokestacks, small factories across the river in Queens, and a cacophony of tugboats belching black effluvia, many of them shouldering against the tide barges that teemed with New York's waste—nothing "belle" about that view at all. Bellevue, with its high ceilings, cavernous rooms, east-west wings jutting from a north-south connector, looked like an ungainly comb straightening an unruly East River. Its inside walls were painted the unhealthy greens and tans of city hospitals everywhere. Its high ceilings held single small bulbs, insufficient to dispel the gloom. Ugly and immense, Bellevue gathered then and gathers now into its ambulance bays, its clinics, and its wards the poor, tired, sick, and hungry, with us now as intensely as they were in Emma Lazarus' day.

In the 1960s Bellevue spoke a dozen languages. It had locked jail wards and tuberculosis wards and psychiatric wards. The jail wards were almost always full, and even on the open floors men and sometimes women were chained to the metal bedsteads, with Department of Corrections officers or city police guards or psychiatric attendants dozing in chairs alongside. Other patients, coughing, consumptive, wandered about the wards with surgical masks, less than token defenses against tuberculosis, dangling ineffectively from an ear. We, the residents, vaguely hoped that these men would not infect fellow patients—or us.

At Bellevue groans and smells and invectives in many tongues assaulted one's senses throughout the day and night. It was the collecting place for the horrors that man inflicts on man: those that he directly inflicts, with guns, knives, needles, and drugs, and those that he indirectly inflicts, with immigration papers, insurance policies, and public laws. At Bellevue I saw patients who waited until the last possible minute to come for help because they were ashamed that they could not pay the bills. I saw a husband of fifty years sell his car, his house, and everything else of value to provide custodial care for a wife disabled by a stroke. I saw couples divorce so that the well, surviving spouse might keep a house and retain some control over a future life alone after the ill one was gone. What I did not see then, but did later, when I rode the police ambulance, and even later when I worked in small mining villages in West Virginia, were the people who chose, even those with treatable diseases, to die unattended because they could not afford care at all. Chances are my uncle, in Mount Vernon, Ohio, never saw such people. He may not even have known of their plight.

Bellevue treated anyone who fell ill within its Manhattan domain—the Bowery and Wall Street, Greenwich Village, the United Nations and the Lower East Side. Bellevue's domain was Chinese and Jewish and Spanish and black and Italian and Greek. But inside its walls, all its beds were alike. There were no private rooms.

One night, we confused the identities of two unconscious men delivered to us, minutes apart, by police ambulances. Both men were in their sixties, tall, white, with identical white hair. Each had an identical stroke paralyzing his left side. Neither could speak. One was a Scandinavian consul at the United Nations, the other a homeless man. Washed, shaved, in hospital johnnies, they looked alike to us. We residents found the situation funny. Members of the Scandinavian consulate, who later arrived, did not share our amusement ("Exactly which one of these gentlemen belongs to you, sir?"). But we treated both as best we could.

The ambulances delivered Wall Street bankers, street drunkards, struggling immigrants, prostitutes, and violent criminals to Bellevue's emergency room. We residents gave no thought to whence the patient came. Or almost no thought. We did note who had lice and who did not. In the pre-AIDS days, lice were nasty mementos of a day in the emergency room that residents could bring home.

What did "the best care we could give" mean to someone hospitalized at Bellevue? It meant, for one thing, that a patient's primary physician was a fourth-year medical student supervised by a new resident, just recently graduated, himself supervised by someone two years more experienced. At Bellevue, in those days, a senior ("attending") physician visited each open ward, with forty or so patients housed together, for an hour, three times a week. The patient had movable screens that he could put around his bed if he used the bedpan, but there were no private rooms, no bedside telephones, no television. There were no beepers for the doctors: overhead paging systems squawked throughout the night.

Our intensive-care area was really a receiving area—a vast room with two rows of beds on one side of a central partition for the men, two rows on the other side for the women. The very sickest patients spent their first days there because this was the only place in the hospital with round-the-clock nursing care. It was a place of neither privacy nor grace.

To those who did not know anything about the underside of New York City, what assaulted the eyes and ears at Bellevue could startle. Example: a dignified, older man, a Wall Street type, collapsed at his office, and the police had brought him to us—a typical heart-attack admission. We had three or four every day. The first few hours of this man's heart attack had been tumultuous. His blood pressure had been dangerously low. His heart rhythm had been erratic. His lungs had filled with fluid. Now, almost a day later, all that was better, but we had not reached the point where we were confident enough of his stability to send him to the conventional-care ward. He was resting, and we residents began to rest, too.

Tant pis, as the French say. Suddenly sirens wailed, puncturing the normal ER cacophony. The ambulances were a block, maybe two blocks away, we guessed from the sound. A moment later flashing lights from the ambulance bay washed the walls in crimson—blink on, off, then on, blink, blink, blink. The double entrance doors crashed open. Two stretchers. Half a dozen police officers. Blood everywhere and much screaming. Gang warfare somewhere south of us, the police said, by way of introduction. Two kids here with multiple gunshot wounds. Maybe more on the way.

One boy was hemorrhaging badly. A bullet in his abdomen must have hit the aorta or the liver. Our surgeons, having heard the sirens, arrived within the instant. No time to ponder here. Bedside anesthesia. Slash with the knife, in with the gloved hand, pinch shut the ruptured artery, then race to the operating room to complete the repair. All this took place in full view of the entire ward, since bedside curtains get in the way of the surgical team. Blood sprayed in jets to the ceiling, onto the walls, and also across the face and chest of my heart-attack patient, bolt upright in bed, mouth gaping open in horror, his heart now tumbled back into the chaotic rhythm we had corrected just half an hour before.

No privacy. No graciousness. Not even dignity, except the dignity of being alive and of being human. But in the end we didn't need the graciousness. Both the boy and my heart-attack patient survived, and that's what counted.

Common courtesy was rare at Bellevue. The kitchen, for instance: it took me nearly a year to realize that when I ordered kosher meals for a patient, Bellevue solved the problem simply by offering no meat on the tray. Or building services: one piercingly cold winter Friday night when the boiler failed and there was no heat, we called hospital maintenance, who referred us to the engineering department of the City of New York, which informed us that it was a weekend. We knew that already. No heating engineers were on call. They would come on Monday, we were told. While we residents pondered, our patients acted: they went to the hall pay telephone (we provided the coins) and called the newly introduced and much vaunted night mayor's hot line. The patients reached the night mayor. An engineer appeared. We had heat by Saturday morning.

Beyond the bricks and mortar and medical students, if you came to Bellevue your health sometimes depended on the health of New York City's finances. Each year we began to run out of antibiotics when the money ran out in March or April, and we could not buy more until the new budget year began in July. Sometimes, to save money, we used outdated drugs—better than using no drugs at all. In that era rich hospitals had the newly invented disposable needles and syringes. They even had butterfly needles—short, small needles with plastic wings—that could be easily inserted and taped down. They had plastic catheters that made it possible to keep intravenous lines in place for days. Bellevue, on the other hand, still used glass syringes and needles that we had to sharpen and sterilize after each use. To the dismay of both patients and residents, because of this old equipment, most of our intravenous lines lasted less than a day. But we tried to compensate. We sent fellow medical students, who rotated to the rich hospitals uptown at other times of the year, to steal the equipment we needed. We thought of it as sharing, because we were all part of the same medical school.

And at Bellevue itself, we were not completely without resources. We were able to do some fancy things, like threading pressure measuring tubes into the heart, as the rich hospitals could do, though only once a week when the uptown specialist visited, not every day. We could inject dye to light up arteries on X-rays when the radiology department had enough dye, when there was enough X-ray film, and when the X-ray machine worked. Because of research done by our professors, we also had the first dialysis service in New York and a Nobel Prize laboratory that had introduced cardiac catheterization to medicine a generation before.

If you were admitted to Bellevue, you were supposed to receive nursing care (you thought). At night, we had one registered nurse to cover sometimes as many as five floors, each floor containing two wards of forty patients each, with only practical nurses and aides as assistants. But only she was authorized to give injections and to put medicines in intravenous infusions. On good nights, we also had one practical nurse or one nursing student to watch over a single ward. Some nights there was only the resident and no nurses at all, meaning that many temperatures and blood-pressure readings were neither taken nor charted.

I do not know if the original patient charts from that era are still available. If so, it would be instructive to look at the "heat sheets"—the graphs that show individual patients' daily fluctuations of pulse, temperature, and blood pressure. You would see many large empty spaces. A few charts would show dutifully recorded measurements of patients who had been released on day passes to attend to personal concerns, and of others who had died. Some aides preferred writing fantasy to walking the wards.

On the nights, weekends, and holidays when there were no floor nurses, the residents mixed the antibiotics and gave the insulin injections themselves. That system was adequate enough, though the residents complained, so long as they did not have to rush to other acutely ill patients in a different part of the hospital. When that happened an injection, or two, or ten, might be skipped. It did not escape our ironic, unspoken notice (we were the "silent generation"; another feeling would be more in vogue today) that very stable diabetics, patients who faithfully and punctually injected themselves with their own insulin at home, usually became unstable when they depended on us.

If you had money and were a patient in one of the uptown hospitals, there were many nurses. There were no antibiotic or X-ray shortages and no forty-bed wards. Medical services were supplied twenty-four hours a day. Attending physicians were available when the residents needed advice. You could buy a great deal of medical care if you could pay. If you could not, the care was there, at Bellevue, just as my uncle said it was, but it was there at a Third World level.

Bellevue still exists, but it is no longer the medieval almshouse it once was. Because of the money that Medicare and Medicaid add to its budget, Bellevue now has two- and four-bed rooms. Attending physicians take responsibility for ward patients. The equipment is modern. Staffing is less of a problem. If you walk into Bellevue today and do not look to see the home addresses of its patients or hear what languages they speak, and if you ignore its prison wards, it will appear no different from other university hospitals.

My uncle's confidence that all was right in the world, that sick people were not abandoned if they could not pay, was not justified in the United States in 1963. My uncle would have been closer to correct had he practiced ten or twenty or thirty years later, when Medicare and Medicaid still provided safety nets for the elderly and for the poor. In the early 1960s there had been a debate on the question: Is health care a right or is it a privilege? In the late 1960s Medicare and Medicaid provided the answer: a right, unquestionably a right. That answer has been true for thirty years.

Today, there is another question: How much are we willing to pay to provide that right? Are there limits to the amount of medical care to which a patient has a right? Is care beyond those limits a privilege? These questions, too, require answers.

As I write, we are all debating the costs of medical care. Some (possessors of the privilege?) consider anew that medical care is an "entitlement," an unearned privilege that often seems excessively generous (to those who do not possess the privilege?), or often a squandering of funds in situations where they can do no good. Perhaps the 1960s' answer should be modified: medical care is a partial, limited right. If those who argue against "entitlement" think only dichotomously—medical care is either a right or a privilege—and do not consider an in-between answer, that it is a partial rationing, a right with limits, and if those who support the "privilege" answer win, the old Bellevue will return, and Dr. Rutstein's assignment to his medical students will be instructive once again.

A LOCAL CITY HOSPITAL

Fred Thomas died on an oppressive, rain-filled day late in the summer of 1963 surrounded by his family. The official record says that a rare heart tumor caused his death, but I think he died of LCH.

That acronym, LCH, had special meaning to me and to my fellow residents at Bellevue. Bellevue was an LCH—a local city hospital. Those three letters, scribbled by a felt-tip pen diagonally across a pink, lined New York City interhospital transfer slip, the slip pinned to the outer clothing of a hapless bearer, LCH assigned the new arrival to Bellevue's emergency room. The hastily scrawled marks indicated indifference and finality. An LCH label was the way in which an uptown hospital had declared that it was not going to help a sick (undesirable) person. It said to us, the residents, "Rejected by a richer hospital."

The way a patient got labeled LCH worked like this: He applied for admission to a private hospital, perhaps because the hospital was near his home or because he respected its reputation. At that hospital's emergency room, on his own authority a resident physician evaluated the patient and decided either to admit him—or to admit him to some other hospital. Or perhaps the hospital administrator made the decision, or the triage nurse. By scrawling the letters LCH on the appropriate piece of paper, no other details necessary, no questions asked or answered, the uptown hospital staff dispatched the patient in a city ambulance (no charge—the city always sent one) to the nearest charity hospital. If the patient complained, the uptown hospital needed only to say, "No beds available." No matter if that was true or untrue, no one would check, or almost no one. Sometimes we, the recipient hospital residents, angry at the callousness, would pretend to be on the staff of an uptown hospital and call its emergency room to inquire about admitting a (fictional) wealthy patient with an interesting disease. No matter which hospital it was that had sent us an "LCH (no beds)" patient, it always had a bed for our fictional patient.

In compassionate translation, the LCH label said to us, "Sick person. We cannot help. Please assume care." But we knew that LCH really said, "Poor. No insurance. May be dirty. May be homeless." Or: "Uninteresting medical problem." Or both. In 1963 the acronym also sometimes said, "Black." Mostly the letters simply meant "Unwanted." But the term LCH was more than an emergency room code used by rich hospitals. At its most grotesque, it denoted the final rung of what we residents termed the Descent of Man: the completed journey—as chronic illness exhausted personal and family resources—of our newly admitted patient from the elegant private suites of the upper floors of the uptown hospitals, to its semiprivate rooms, then to its ward service, and finally, when nothing remained, to the LCH.

Fred Thomas had followed this route. In health, he had been hardworking, kind, devout, and conscientious. These traits were evident when he fell ill. He was not rich when illness forced him to stop working, nor was he poor, but he died a pauper. The illness care system had consumed it all.

My fellow residents and I received this gentle man on our floor, LCH'd with a diagnosis of end-stage heart disease and no insurance. As admitting residents always do, we evaluated him again, partly because we were careful doctors and partly because it was a joy to find something undiscovered, to prove that we were better doctors than the ones uptown. In Mr. Thomas' case we did find something. We detected a medically interesting illness, a rare heart tumor, surgically curable. Armed with this new diagnosis, we first telephoned the uptown doctors who had LCH'd him to gloat, then we hunted for ways to subvert the system. Mr. Thomas' illness now enticed the other doctors to help, and as a result we gained access for him to a patchwork assemblage of advanced medical care beyond what Bellevue could provide. We found someone at the uptown hospital willing to do the critical diagnostic test free of charge. We found a surgeon at a third hospital willing to operate for no fee. But the care we contrived for Mr. Thomas, and were unable to assemble for patients with more prosaic diseases, was, in the end, amateurish and too late.

It was hot and raining on that Monday night. Mr. Thomas had had his surgery at the end of the preceding week at a hospital in Queens where I had never been. I had been on duty throughout the weekend, but now I was free until Tuesday morning. Guided by the map at my side, itself barely visible under the dim Volkswagen map light, peering through fogged windows, I found the hospital in Queens. Visiting hours had ended. But I wore my white Bellevue uniform, and no one stopped me at the door. A nurse directed me to his room.

In the two or three weeks since I had last seen Mr. Thomas, he had aged. He was confused. He could not see. The surgeons had told me that the tumor had shattered when they tried to remove it. Pieces of it had spread to his kidneys and to his brain. His kidneys had ceased to work. Mr. Thomas' daughter and son, at his bedside, told him that I had come. He did not know at first who I was. Then he remembered, and he seemed pleased. I wished him well. He was tired and wanted to sleep. I could see that he would not live.

The next day his daughter paged me from my morning rounds. Her father, she said, had just died. She wanted me to know. The rain continued, that day and the next, until the day of his funeral. But I was on call and I could not go.

In 1963, Fred Thomas' medical care was rationed by his ability to pay. A generation has passed since Fred Thomas died, and

we ration health care for different reasons now—sometimes
on the basis of medical futility, and sometimes on the basis
of society's, not the patient's, inability to pay. Poverty's prox-
ies—no insurance, foreign birth, economic unfeasibility (this
procedure or that drug is not "cost-effective")—are cited as
other reasons to deny care.

These are no improvement on the LCH. Today there are
many people who still cannot obtain medical care. Today policymakers do not ask the advice of these people, even though
they are the ones who most suffer from policy changes. Yet
the chronically ill, the poor, the weak do have a voice. The
voice is soft, and we must make an effort to listen. The needs
of these people must be known.

CHANGING TIMES

Four entities participate in medical-care transactions having
to do with sick patients: an ill person, a medical-care professional, a health-care institution, and a payer. In 1963 the words
that described these entities were: supplicant, altruist, benev-
olent institution, and insurance or bank account or charity.
Other words were not used: choice, dialogue, partnership,
man's responsibility to one's fellow man. There were no
"rights" for a sick person, who had no voice and could not
overrule an LCH label. Patients were rarely partners in their
own care.

Both the science and the sociology of medicine in 1963 appear strange to today's eyes. Forty-two percent of our nation
smoked. Young men died in epidemic proportions from heart
attacks. And, something barely mentioned in any colloquy today, a sixty-five-year-old was old. In 1970, according to the
Census Bureau, less than 10 percent of the population was

more than sixty-five, and life expectancy was less than seventy years. The first nontoxic antibiotic to be effective against the feared hospital bacterium *Staphylococcus aureus*, "yellow staph," had just arrived, and doctors were giddy about its possibilities. Soon all infections will be conquered, we thought—and this was fifteen years before the advent of AIDS. Not even the most gloomy physicians would then have predicted its future pandemic outbreak. Was your medical case puzzling? A specialist physician, preferably one known as a "diagnostician," could solve the problem. Specialists were in high demand. Chemotherapy for cancer was barely known. Polio and smallpox were still extant. If your heartbeat was not right, doctors could pace your heart by administering electric shocks from outside the chest, though not from inside. There were no CAT scans, MRIs, or ultrasound. Dialysis for kidney failure was scarcely available outside research hospitals. Even in those hospitals there were "God committees" that selected candidates for dialysis according to rules that assessed one's eligibility according to some measure of one's communal worth. Cardiac and medical intensive-care units had not yet been invented. There were very few effective drugs for treating high blood pressure. Patients with chronic and crippling illnesses lived, often without their consent, on the wards of chronic-disease hospitals or in state psychiatric institutions. No one but doctors knew the word "cholesterol." Syphilis, the most feared venereal disease and a cause for deep shame, was discussed in whispers and people used euphemisms for it, like "bad blood," but it was curable. There were no neonatal intensive-care units; premature babies mostly died; even the scarcely premature (by today's standards) child of the President of the United States could not be saved. Legal abortions were very rare, and illegal ones were commonplace. I vividly remember a frightened twenty-two-year-old victim of a back-alley abor-

tion, far from home, accompanied by her equally terrified boy-
friend, whom we sent for an emergency hysterectomy at
midnight and then for weeks treated with dialysis for kidney
failure. She lingered at death's door for a month. The irony
was that she was an exchange student from a country famous
(or infamous) for its legal abortion policy. Had she been able
to afford the trip, she could have gone home, where abortions
were legal and safe.

In 1963, you purchased what medical care you could afford.
The very rich could, to extraordinary degrees, command America's best medical resources. One immensely rich lady spent
years as an inpatient in a private room in an elegant hospital,
using the room as a hotel because she preferred neither to go
to a nursing home nor to remain bedridden at home. (This
bored the hospital residents immensely. As they rotate to different tours of duty, they normally write supposedly matter-
of-fact "on-service" notes in the charts of patients they are
just meeting and "off-service" notes in the charts of those
whom they leave. The residents responsible for the lady in
question vied to write, in a more original way than their pre-
decessors, "Nothing happened on my tour." Copies of the
notes circulated among them like a sort of underground humor
magazine.) Another wealthy woman in another hospital got
herself two adjoining rooms, hired carpenters to punch a door
through the wall between, and set up a suite for her husband
and her own private chef, for a hospital stay of about six weeks.
When she went home, the door was sealed over, but its outline
remained visible for years.

If you were too poor to buy much medical care, and if your
savings were gone, you might still find some high-tech medicine at your local charity hospital, despite its forty-bed open
wards and its nursing and medication shortages. Medical
schools supplied its equipment and physicians; the city gave

the bricks and mortar and sometimes the heat and the nurses and maintenance personnel. There was no Medicare or Medicaid, and there certainly were no Health Maintenance Organizations.

In short, the discrepancies between care for the rich and care for the poor were enormous. In 1963 the United States needed more doctors, more specialists, more medical schools, more hospitals, and more medical research. Magazines, newspapers, congressional committees, and doctors' committees all said so. State and federal governments attempted to ease the scarcities. Saturation quantities of cash came in the form of hospital capital grants, medical-school foundings, medical-school capitation grants, and federal research grants. And the policies worked.

Between 1960 and 1990, the number of medical schools grew 57 percent, the number of medical students 114 percent, medical-school faculties 526 percent, while the population grew only 38 percent.* In 1970 there were 15 physicians for every 10,000 Americans; by 1996, this number was 24, an increase of 60 percent. Between 1970 and 1995 federal expenditures for medical research, in constant dollars, grew 280 percent.

Yet there continued to be a cry for more medical specialists. Specialists, after all, had the latest tools and the best information to cure disease. The needs of patients were not being met, people and doctors agreed. In the 1970s, I headed a crash program to increase the teaching of rheumatology in medical schools. My committee noted that one-quarter of America's medical schools had no rheumatology staff at all. We worried,

*See E. H. Ahrens, *The Crisis in Clinical Medicine* (New York, 1992), and U.S. Bureau of the Census, *Statistical Abstract of the United States: 1995 and 1997.*

with reason, that people seeking care from graduates of these schools would be poorly served. Every school needed a training program in each specialty, we said, each program graduating three or four new specialists each year. We focused on the future in times of want, and we could not foresee a day when there would be an oversupply.

Americans who had medical insurance did not consider medical care expensive in the 1960s. If a technology was available to sustain life, *and if the person could afford it*, then that technology was applied. There was rationing, a lot of it, but it was rationing on the basis of the patient's wealth. "Cost-effectiveness," "gatekeeper," "limited resources": these concepts simply were not part of public discourse. But there also were no coronary bypass procedures, PET scans, heart transplants, surviving one-and-a-half-pound babies, or other evidence of highly expensive medical procedures. Very few people were eighty years old, so there was little Alzheimer's disease. The circumstances in which a single patient, even in a very short time, might cost an insurer's entire budget were rare. No one talked about keeping people alive against their wishes. We doctors would not have known how.

1

PATIENTS AND THEIR DOCTORS

PARTNERS

Chances are that you don't think about your doctor very much, or consult him often about day-to-day things you want to do, because most likely your only contact with him has been for an acute, probably short-term illness or injury. But many among us suffer from chronic long-term diseases. Those of us who do enter into a form of partnership with our physicians. Like a marriage, this is a true partnership—no dominant partner, no submissive partner—just two people, physician and patient, working out acceptable solutions for a problem. Small and large decisions, the trivia of daily life, are the currency of their transactions. Can I eat this? Is it okay for me to visit my sister in Pittsburgh? Do you know a doctor in Omaha? Would a glass of champagne hurt me at my son's wedding? In chronic illness, the partners negotiate the treatments. Long-range goals take precedence over immediate problems. The telephone is an important resource.

As a doctor caring for patients with chronic illness, I commonly perform what I call a physical examination by telephone. If a family member of a patient calls to tell me that my patient has a fever, or some other minor complaint, I insist on talking directly to the patient. My purpose is not to be difficult but to hear the strength of the patient's voice and the worry in the vocal tone. Because of our partnership, I know my patient well enough to make an accurate judgment, on the basis of my telephone observation, about how urgent the problem is. (I have not mastered the art of diagnosing rashes over the telephone. No one commands a vocabulary sufficient for that task.)

With Medicare and Medicaid, this partnership occurs whether the patient lives on Park Avenue or in Harlem. There are not two sets of rules, one for the rich and one for the poor, as there was when I was in medical school. I do not—my hospital does not—refuse to hospitalize a Medicaid patient because she is poor, and I do not hospitalize a privately insured patient for her personal convenience because she is rich. Some of our hospital rooms are more elegant than others, of course, but admission is determined by the illness, not by the method of payment. Is the patient sick enough to take our last available bed? the admitting office asks, not What kind of insurance does he have? At times, when the hospital is very crowded, any patient—Medicaid or privately insured—can go to any room; there are a few surprised roommates when Park Avenue meets the Bowery.

Before Medicare and Medicaid, then after, poor and rich patients with chronic illness had different fates.

One day in the mid-1960s, Bellevue's admitting officer called to tell me that Mabel McDougal was headed to my floor. Self-absorbed, like most medical residents, I mostly hoped that hers would be a simple admission, which usually took about two hours of work. I averaged about four admissions each time I was on call. Long charts about a prior hospitalization, or a patient with a complex illness destroyed whatever organization I hoped to impose upon my day. It turned out that Mabel McDougal had a short prior chart, only two volumes deep, and, *mirabile dictu*, it actually preceded her to the floor. (Bellevue's medical records department won no prizes for efficiency in those days.)

The chart gave me the essential details: Ms. McDougal had systemic lupus erythematosus. She had been admitted to Bellevue several times before because of fever, inflammation of the membrane that lines the heart, arthritis, and other symptoms typical of lupus. Her symptoms this time were the same. The disease had flared. She wasn't super-sick. It was just a matter of readjusting her medications again—easy to do and done in a few days. Quick admission. Better than I feared.

There was a problem. It was not that her illness had recurred or that she had had to be admitted again. Both were straight-forward enough, almost commonplace. The problem was that I was her doctor.

I don't say that to denigrate my own skills, though my skills were certainly modest. But Ms. McDougal had been ill for three years and she had no personal doctor. Instead, her doctor was the medical resident assigned to the female medicine ward, whoever that might be. Off and on for the three years of my residency, two months of the year on the ward and five in outpatient clinic, I had been that doctor. When I was as-signed to an affiliated hospital, her doctor was someone else (except when I—shading the truth about her abnormal blood counts—sneaked her onto the cancer service at my new hospital). When I went into military service for two years in the middle of my Bellevue service, Ms. McDougal saw a different resident, but when I came back, I was her doctor again. So her medical chart, available only at random intervals, was the only constant factor in her care. She had little to say about all of this, because she was poor. She could choose among the other available city (charity) hospitals in our district, but private hospitals were beyond her reach. When I completed my residency and went to another hospital in New York, I lost contact with her forever.

In those pre-Medicare days, hospital emergency rooms posted local area maps near the entrance desk. Red lines marked the perimeters of the hospital's obligation. Was the patient found, or did he reside, within the red lines? If so, he was eligible for care here, but if he came from outside the line, was not immediately dying, and could not pay, he had to go to the charity hospital responsible for that district.

Then the world changed. Medicare and Medicaid gave poor patients control over their medical lives—empowered them, to use today's phrase, to select their own care. When I moved once again to one of the rich uptown hospitals, I invited my poor clinic patients to come with me. Uptown hospitals now accepted poor patients so long as they had Medicaid. And if they didn't, no problem: the hospital would apply to Medicaid for them. The red-lined maps still hang in the emergency rooms. But now the red lines are there only to direct ambulances and police cars calling in about patients they hope to transport. The maps are irrelevant to patients who arrive on their own at our doors. For that matter, the maps are irrelevant to the ambulance drivers, since they need not follow the emergency room's advice.

———

Tia Hendricks showed me how empowerment works. Street-wise, very independent at the age of sixteen, she was ill with lupus and first hospitalized near her home, at Kings County Hospital, the Brooklyn LCH. This was after Medicaid was enacted, rather than before.

The doctors at Kings County told Ms. Hendricks they wanted to perform a kidney biopsy to assess the health of her kidneys. In those days there were two ways to do a biopsy. The old, time-honored way was a surgical operation: the patient undergoes full anesthesia, the surgeon makes a four-inch incision in the flank through which he reaches in to remove a small piece of kidney. The surgery takes about an hour (three if you count anesthesia time) and recovery about a week. Because the surgeon cuts muscles that participate in one's breathing, recovering patients hurt with each breath and whenever they move, a pain that lasts for several days, with unpleasant twinges continuing for weeks. The other way, with local anesthesia and an X-ray, doctors guide a small biopsy needle through the skin; this takes about an hour (the actual use of the needle takes only a few minutes), and is much less painful—the patient gets out of bed a few hours later and goes home the next day. At Kings County Hospital, Ms. Hendricks' roommate had just had a surgical kidney biopsy done and was crying with pain. Ms. Hendricks asked her doctors about alternatives. She learned about the needle biopsy, not then available at that hospital, made a few telephone calls, and learned that our hospital did do the needle biopsy. Though she still was not certain she would consent to any biopsy, surgical or needle, she signed herself out of Kings County and took the subway to us in mid-Manhattan.

"They ain't cuttin' on me," she said, her Kings County identification bracelet still tightly encircling her wrist. "Can you
treat me?" She wore a gang-insignia leather jacket and jeans—
a statement in those days. A cigarette dangled from the corner
of her mouth. But her street bravado and language did not
successfully mask her wide eyes and tentative speech. Barely
five feet tall, under one hundred pounds, she was still a
sixteen-year-old, sick, and alone (though not as alone as she
first seemed, since her parents eventually found out where she
was and joined her at our clinic). Ms. Hendricks was neither
articulate nor well educated, but her request was clear.

The answer to her question was of course yes. We needed
her parents' permission because, despite her tough-kid appearance, she was a minor—but she was sick, our clinic was
expert in her problem, and we could treat her because Medicaid paid, not enough to support private hospitals like ours
fully, but enough to allow us to treat poor patients like her
without risking bankruptcy.

For Ms. Hendricks and for me, our brief conversation was
conclusive. Though we came from worlds as far apart as they
could be, in that moment we formed a close partnership, close
enough so that I later shared the joy of her wedding and still
later was godfather to her child. When minor things happened—an injury, a bout of flu, a family crisis, something wonderful her daughter did—she was as comfortable calling me to
discuss it as were any of my rich private patients. We were
partners in her care.

It was still a close partnership when she died, a decade or
so later, of complications from lupus. On her deathbed, her
voice so weak that I had to bend my ear to her lips to hear,
her words coming in twos and threes as she gasped for breath,
she asked me to hold her hand, and I did. She then asked me
to take a package from her bedside cabinet drawer. It con-

tained an enlarged, framed photograph of her daughter. She gave me the picture and asked me to protect her child after she was gone.

Ms. McDougal and Ms. Hendricks fell victim to lupus only a few years apart. Neither was well educated. Both were poor. In most respects they were very alike, even to the specifics of their disease. Ms. McDougal glanced off first one doctor, then another, never had a telephone number to call to discuss the trivia of her daily life, never knew who would fill her next prescription. Ms. McDougal had no partner in her care, but Ms. Hendricks did. Since I was the doctor for both, I know that I didn't make the difference. The difference was the empowerment Medicaid gives to patients, the government's safety net for the weak, the government granting patients with chronic illness a measure of dignity in and control over their own lives.

UGLIES

All doctors know about the uglies. They are not much talked about, but go onto any hospital ward, certainly into any nursing home, and you will see the uglies. They cause more misery than almost any other medical problem, though as a rule people do not die from them, or talk about them.

In a hospital or a nursing home, you know the uglies are there because you smell them. You see a certain lack of enthusiasm, sometimes masked revulsion, on the faces of the doctors and nurses when they enter certain rooms. The uglies are socially and aesthetically unsuitable symptoms that happen to decent human beings. Biology has no social or aesthetic sense. The uglies are skin ulcers, bedsores, and incontinence. They are awful for people. They are expensive. A single bedsore may cost $40,000 to heal.*

Nobody likes the uglies, but they are there, as much a part of medicine as cancer, heart attack, or stroke. And treating them is an important part of medical care.

Despite the bright spring sunshine, Keisha Franklin's room was dark. The shades were drawn, because her inflamed eyes burned in bright light. She was in misery from this and from many other problems.

The medical resident wanted to introduce me to Ms. Franklin, but Ms. Franklin showed no pleasure in meeting me. Her first words were not those most people deem polite. I do not want to quote her precisely—you will understand if I say that she proffered, with strong emotion and short Anglo-Saxon words, vivid thoughts on both animal physiology and my parentage. The opinions she volunteered about me were not those that tend to strengthen fellowship.

It would be fair to say that she was not herself that day. High fever and uncontrollable vomiting could not add to her good humor. She was in severe pain. She thought her insides were aflame: her pancreas, tired of the insults it had daily received from illegal drugs and alcohol, was disgorging enzymes that, unchecked, would digest her body from the inside out. All these symptoms were worse because she was withdrawing from cocaine and/or heroin addiction, I'm not sure which—

*K. J. Inman, W. J. Sibbald, F. S. Rutledge, and B. J. Clark, "Clinical Utility and Cost-Effectiveness of an Air Suspension Bed in the Prevention of Pressure Ulcers," *Journal of the American Medical Association*, 1993, 269: 1139–43.

the details were fuzzy at the time. She had lupus, as well. The lupus in turn had caused two of the largest and nastiest leg ulcers I had ever seen or smelled. The ulcers oozed odious and fetid muck from flesh that, from knees to ankles, had rotted away. The ulcers would have looked excessive in a Bosch painting. Baudelaire, in his blackest mood, would not have known what to say.

Ms. Franklin arrived at our hospital—by what means I did not find out—with no reference from a personal doctor. An administrator had decided that the diagnosis of lupus outranked her other diagnoses and assigned her care to me.

Ms. Franklin's inflamed pancreas, her drug addiction, and her accompanying infections were routine problems for me and my medical team. The lupus and her social activities— drug selling as well as drug using, prostitution, a home the existence of which was at best vague—were more challenging but also within our experience. She did not have the AIDS virus, an encouraging point. Her decidedly negative reaction to me did not matter so much. Even if she had wanted to, Ms. Franklin was too ill to go to another hospital. For my part, I was not of the school that says that doctors have to like or be liked by all their patients. As it happened, after the first outburst she was too exhausted to contest my assuming her care. And anyway it wasn't likely that she'd like another doctor better. She did not fire me, not then and not over the next several years.

We took care of the immediate problems first, which responded well to treatment. Then the leg ulcers dominated both my attention and hers. In theory, it is a simple matter to heal a leg ulcer: keep it immaculately clean and free of infection, protect it from injury, maintain the surrounding tissue in as healthy a condition as possible, treat fastidiously the underlying disease, and apply a skin graft if necessary. It will heal.

But it takes months at the very least, and it is hard for both doctors and patients to be consistently meticulous over such an extended time. Many ulcers never heal.

We doctors tend to celebrate our rare triumphs with large and long-standing ulcers. When another patient of mine, much richer than Ms. Franklin, tended to by her husband and supported by an army of visiting nurses, healed one over many months, we—she, her husband, I, and another physician— drank champagne. Another triumph was George Penney. He had been bed-bound for more than two years with rheumatoid arthritis, and he had had ulcers on both ankles for at least as long. Mr. Penney's joints were permanently bent. Hips, knees, elbows, and feet at right angles, hands, wrists, shoulders, and ankles frozen in place, he was as incapacitated as it is possible to be. His teenage daughter fed, bathed, and helped him with his toilet needs (his wife had long since left). And then she brought him to us. He wanted to walk again. Neither he nor his daughter expected to heal the ulcers. Painful and distasteful as they were, he would live with them if he could walk.

We doctors saw the problem differently. We could not fix his destroyed joints because infection in the ulcers would infect the artificial joints we wanted to use. So we called in collaborators who were testing new methods of healing skin ulcers. They accepted Mr. Penney onto their research ward, his costs to be paid by their research grant. It took more than a year, but my colleagues healed the ulcers. Then we brought Mr. Penney back to our hospital to replace his joints. He walked out of the hospital holding his daughter's arm—a scene from a wedding that was not a wedding, father and daughter both radiating pride in the accomplishment. The doctors, researchers, clinicians, and surgeons radiated equal pride.

Ms. Franklin's leg ulcers were worse than those of Mr. Penney, in fact so bad that we discussed amputating her legs. Since she could not eat during the two months it took her pancreas to heal (we fed her intravenously), she stayed in the hospital, and four times we took her to the operating room to cut dead tissue from her legs; other times we removed dead tissue at the bedside. (To do that we gave large doses of narcotics, notwithstanding her former addiction, to control the pain.)

Her nutrition improved. The lupus quieted down. As she felt better, her mood lightened. We saw her humor. She daily ridiculed the failings of her medical-care team—us—but she had wit, and she criticized us with a smile. Over these weeks the barriers between Ms. Franklin and me eased. We talked. We talked about the leg ulcers, about the impediments to healing that her personal life imposed. She told me I didn't know her: if she put her mind to it, she said, she could heal the ulcers. We made a pact: she would prove to me that she could stay off drugs and heal the ulcers; I promised her that I would treat her to a dinner for two at a fashionable restaurant when the ulcers healed. I thought it would take years.

Two years later Ms. Franklin enjoyed that dinner. Her sister was her guest. That gave me double pleasure, because her sister also had lupus; she now trusted me enough to bring her sister to me for help. I did not join them at the dinner, but I know that they were suitable customers in that stylish place; with healing and with civil treatment, Ms. Franklin had gained transforming self-respect, and I knew the strength of that transformation.

When I left New York some of my patients held a goodbye party for me. Some gave me personal gifts. Ms. Franklin's was the best. Well dressed, standing tall, voice clear and strong, she recited a poem she had written, the verses structured around the letters of my name. The poem was embarrassingly loving. As she read, I thought of the day we first met, and tears came to my eyes. They still do.*

What is the lesson of Ms. Franklin's story? It is not her personal growth, though that is important. It is that continuous and diligent care, improvement measured in minute increments, has value to individual patients. Ms. Franklin gained self-esteem when she healed her legs. That was not high-tech medical care. There were no expensive machines or state-of-the-art science interventions. Just a physician and a patient working together over an extended time.

At what cost? Not so much, really, except that the care given to Ms. Franklin fit no definition of efficiency. Her initial hospitalization was too long by contemporary standards. (Mr. Penney's hospitalization, even though paid for by a research protocol, would be intolerable in today's HMO or Medicaid or utilization-committee standards.) My wealthy patient could afford to pay for her visiting nurse visits; Medicare would have covered far fewer.

Are skin ulcers to be ignored, then? Skin ulcers are ugly. One does not discuss them in polite company. Because they are unpleasant, they get little public attention. But if we talked more about them publicly we'd understand that these and other "small ticket" issues cause enormous distress. The uglies exist whether we want them to or not, and to the afflicted patients the uglies are very real. They require extensive phy-

---

*Self-respect, dignity, and pride are fragile things. The doctor who assumed her care had a different style than did I and was more rigid in his rules. Ms. Franklin drifted away from the clinic, returned to her former lifestyle, and died of AIDS a few years later.

sician and nursing time, not high-tech tools, and they do not stand out as "must reimburse" on the list of most health-care payers' priorities. A baboon-to-human transplant will make national news, but raising the success rate of skin-ulcer healing will not. Skin ulcers are not part of our national conversation.

A medical-care system that purports to be fair must help the Keisha Franklins and the George Penneys just as it helps those with more dramatic disease. To those with uglies, to those suffering from chronic illness, slow and incremental gains have value. Dignity has value. Self-image has value. Relief from pain has value. Walking, and using the toilet unassisted, have value. These values are as important and lifesaving as coronary bypass surgery. Comfort and independence at even minimal levels have value.

SLAVES AND SLAVEMASTERS

Darlene Jamison bit the nurse, slugged an aide, and grabbed my arm so hard that I had bruises for weeks. Small, a little overweight, she did not at first glance look very strong, but terror enhances strength. She seemed afraid—of what we did not know. Her wild glances from side to side, the occasional intelligible words she screamed, gave us no clues. There were no imaginary people in the room. It was we who frightened her. Alone, or with her mother, she was calm, but with us she screamed, bit the nurse, slugged an aide, and bruised my arm.

During her brief lucid moments she would tell us that she really is a very nice person, cheerful all the time. Her mother would tell us this, too. She'd be embarrassed by what the staff told her she had done. But after an hour or so the delirium would begin again. To treat her we put her in restraints. (That is a euphemism. What we did was tie her to her bed with leather straps around her arms and legs, a tough canvas binder around her stomach, and sedate her.) She struggled hard against the straps. They left burn marks on her skin.

A combination of high fever, lupus, and cortisone had caused delirium. Her situation was worse than it might have been. Her doctors had made the correct diagnosis and initially had treated her correctly. But within a week Ms. Jamison had become hyperactive, euphoric, too talkative, insomniac. These are common side effects of the cortisone treatment; they could have been lupus symptoms as well. When unsure which, experienced doctors administer tranquilizers to calm the patient and continue the cortisone. Instead, Ms. Jamison's doctors reduced the dose, whereupon her high fever and pain returned. They increased the cortisone again. She became agitated, then delirious. They decreased the cortisone. Active lupus again. Seesaw drug doses and seesaw disease. At that point they asked us to assume Ms. Jamison's care.

To control severe lupus, it is necessary to continue high-dose cortisone for several weeks whether a patient is delirious or not. If necessary, sedate and tranquilize the patient, but continue the drug. We followed the conventional rule. We kept the dose high, sedated her (tied her to her bed), and waited for the drug to take effect. Day by day her fright lessened. She was very confused for a few days, then tearful, then less confused, then calm. We removed the restraints. Within a few weeks Ms. Jamison was thinking normally. We stopped the sedation. We saw that she is a very nice person, cheerful most of the time.

These events took place more than fourteen years ago. Her illness remained difficult, with many complications. She and I have talked often in those fourteen years. We have talked about her life and her future when she married. We talked more when she divorced. We talked about her job. I moved to Maryland, but we stayed in touch. Sometimes she called because there was a problem. Sometimes she called just to tell me things were going well. She called when she won $50,000 in a lottery. She comes to see me as a patient about once a year now, to say hello or to ask me to mediate a disagreement with or among her current doctors. Ms. Jamison's grandmother became ill, then her mother, and we talked about this. Her kidneys failed. She had problems with dialysis. She waited for a kidney transplant. All these things she shared with me.

Eventually she got a new kidney. Recovered from the surgery, excited, she came to show me how well she was now. I watched as she walked toward my examining room. She had gained some weight, which was good—she had been gaunt. Her energy level was high. To me, that day, she looked great. It was obvious that I thought so, and that made her very happy. She kissed me, there, in the waiting room, at the clinic desk. The kiss was not just a social peck; she threw her arms around me and hugged me. She took a camera from her purse and asked the clerk at the desk to take a picture of us together, my arm around her shoulder, her head on my shoulder. She felt truly good.

I was a little nonplussed, and when I get that way I babble. Babbling, I explained to the clerk, who had watched all this, that I had known Darlene Jamison for years and that I could even remember the day we met. Ms. Jamison interrupted: she remembered that day, too. That was a surprise for me. I assumed that because of her delirium she would have no recall of that time at all.

She laughed and asked, "Do you know why I was so frightened of you?"

"No," I answered. "I knew you were frightened, but I didn't know you were frightened *of me*."

Matter-of-factly she replied, "I thought I was a runaway

slave. And you"—she meant the whole medical staff, all of us white, I now suppose, though I no longer remember who was there—"were slavemasters. I thought you were trying to capture me."

Of course.

The day we met, when she bit the nurse and bruised my arm, I unimaginatively had seen only a very sick, delirious young woman—not the very sick, delirious, young *black* woman she was. I had not seen an army of *white* medical personnel. That day, fourteen years ago, I had been a technical doctor, a biologist doctor, but not more. "Runaway slave." I had not seen the world through her eyes.

When a patient enters an examining room, he brings with him a personal story. The doctor, on the other side of the desk, has another. Two persons, doctor and patient, two stories. I am not talking about the medical events. The stories I mean are the stories of families, of social classes, of education, of peoples, of nations, of all sorts of things. Personal stories create bonds between people and barriers too. To draw a conclusion on the basis of what is first seen is to miss an opportunity to understand. I had written in Darlene Jamison's chart, the day we met, what had seemed important to me: "twenty-eight-year-old black woman, computer analyst, single, has been ill for three weeks." I thought then that those demographic identifiers told me something important about her, but I now saw they had told me little, because I had not looked at the world through her eyes. To comprehend, not just to know, who a Darlene Jamison is, to talk with rather than to her, takes work, and imagination that goes beyond the biology of her illness.

"Runaway slave."

"Slavemaster."

Those words, now casually offered by a happy, fairly healthy black woman, showed me, and in doing so removed, a barrier to which I had been blind.

SPECIALISTS, EXPERIENCE, JUDGMENT CALLS

"Mike," my colleague called to me as I raced by him late one Thursday afternoon. I skidded to a stop. "A former classmate of mine just called," he said. "He has a patient, in a small hospital in Connecticut, who sounds pretty sick. He asked me to consult. I told him you go out there on weekends and that you would take a look for me when you go. Is that okay?"

It was okay. The hospital was more than half the way to our house in the country, where my family and I went as often as we could on the weekends when I was not on call. To be sure, we hadn't planned to be there on the coming weekend. I thought I might be able to run up on the Saturday, though. It was only forty-five minutes away, so I called the doctor in Connecticut. He sounded anxious, so I agreed to go on Friday instead. I arranged to meet him at the hospital, late, after the evening rush hour had cleared.

I had not listened to the weather forecast.

On Friday afternoon snow began to fall, a miserable cusp-of-freezing snow, slushy, slippery, neither liquid nor solid. Still, I had made a promise. After rush hour I headed north. I started on the Merritt Parkway, then switched to the New England Thruway, then to back roads, as snow fell and stuck cars blocked the road. I had a four-wheel-drive jeep, but the jeep was not a tank. It could not climb over the other cars or go through the woods that blocked my route. The drive took an hour and a half, maybe more.

Hubert Steiner's family waited for me. His doctor had also

waited, then had gone home, leaving a telephone number for me. I called. I said he needn't come back, but I'd be glad if he did.

Mr. Steiner's eyes met mine when I entered the room. He was a big man, completely filling the hospital bed. Graying, angular, he looked like the corporate executive that his chart told me he was. He lay on his left side facing the door. The family members stood behind or sat in chairs placed so not to block his view.

He had been well, except for asthma, until a few weeks before. First came fever, then his muscles ached. He started to lose strength and feeling in his arms and legs, one body site at a time. Without warning he found that he could not cock his wrist; his hand just flopped. The same thing happened to a foot. The foot became numb. The other foot lost power, the other hand, and the upper arms. Now, in less than a week, he could move neither arm nor either leg.

I asked him to repeat his story again. I know it irks patients when doctors ask the same questions over again, but doctors have different asking styles; they emphasize different things. Patients remember new facts. A specific turn of phrase, a grimace, a pause, body language, each adds something that may not have been noted before. Stopping for breath between phrases, Mr. Steiner tolerantly answered each of my questions. I uncovered little that was new. Mrs. Steiner had kept a diary of her husband's illness. The narrative was pretty complete.

Muscle wasting had already begun, leaving hollows between the tendons on the back of the hand, no flesh in the fleshy part above the thumb, and a concavity where the base of the thumb should have been convex. "Move your leg," I asked him, and I watched. Nothing, not a twitch. "Move your arms, or hands, or fingers." Again nothing. He could shrug one shoulder. He could turn his head. He could talk (one phrase at a time). That was about it.

Our body's nerves are of two main types, and each type has two main jobs. One type is central, the nerves in the brain and spinal cord. The other type is peripheral, nerves that go to the muscles and skin. The jobs are to control muscle motion (motor nerves) or tell you of pain (sensory nerves). Faced with patients like Mr. Steiner, the doctor has to figure out which nerves are injured and why.

I looked first at the nerves of the face (eyes, tongue, ears, smile and frown), neck, and shoulders. One of Mr. Steiner's eyes did not move fully to one side. The bad eye turned upward instead. I had already seen his right shoulder shrug. He could not shrug his left. He could feel a brush and a pin that I lightly touched to his face. I asked him to bend his leg, straighten his leg, lift his arm, squeeze his fist. Just one thigh muscle moved, not enough to raise the leg. Some fingers in his right hand worked. I tested with the pin and brush. Scattered areas had no feeling at all. Other areas were normal. With my rubber-tipped hammer I tapped the reflex points on his knees, ankles, elbows, and wrists, but nothing jumped back. Only his brain seemed untouched by this disease. His thought and speech were normal. His mood was calm, though how he stayed (outwardly) tranquil was a mystery to me.

The pattern was that of injury to many motor and sensory nerves. The damage had occurred in a series of abrupt episodes and was not symmetrical. That pattern, that sequence, has only a few causes. Lead poisoning is one, but there was no reason to think he had that. In any event, a test for lead had been normal. Diabetes is another cause, but Mr. Steiner was not diabetic. Polyarteritis nodosa is a third cause. Mr. Steiner's doctor had done a biopsy to test for this. The results were positive. That is why he had called my colleague.

Polyarteritis nodosa, PAN—medicalese meaning many (poly) inflamed (-itis) and lumpy (nodosa) arteries (arter-)— is a rare disease in which arteries throughout the body become inflamed and blocked. PAN causes many different symptoms, depending on which arteries are inflamed. Block the arteries that nourish peripheral nerves and the nerves die; without the nerves the muscles do not work. Mr. Steiner's condition was the result.

My colleague and I had written some medical papers about PAN. Reading them, other doctors had referred more patients to us, and thus I had cared for many patients with this rare disease. About half of them had died—an average rate of success, I'm sorry to say. If a single clot blocks an artery to a vital organ, like the heart, death can occur even before treatment begins. I was not optimistic.

Stomping snow from his feet, Mr. Steiner's doctor arrived. I chatted briefly with him in private, then together we walked back to talk to the family. Mr. Steiner's doctor asked me to speak first. To do this, I composed myself in a suitably grim way. Doctors do that sometimes—self-consciously pose when talking to strangers—to be certain that they do not convey the wrong message. I was not going to give good news. It was appropriate that my bearing agree with my words.

I sat down in front of Mr. Steiner, deliberately low to look into his eyes. I began by telling him that I agreed with his doctor, that he did have polyarteritis nodosa, and that his case was very severe. "I'm not sure," I went on, staying bleak, "that you will ever walk, or at least walk normally, again." In my peripheral vision I saw his wife, then his children, become restless. I glanced up. I saw smiles!

I wasn't *that* tired, I thought. I did a quick inventory of my own brain to check that my senses were intact. I looked out the window. In the halos around the parking-lot lights I saw that the snow had stopped. Friday night, snowstorm, small Connecticut hospital—it all seemed to fit. It did not seem to be a dream. Yet I was giving a horrible prognosis, and the family seemed cheered by my words.

Uncomprehendingly, I forged ahead. I spoke about the months, perhaps years, that I foresaw for his recovery. I mentioned future complications which could be lethal. I spoke about side effects of the drugs I would use. I said I wanted to transfer him to our big hospital in New York.

Another furtive glance up. The faces were not ambiguous. Their elation had increased. Ordinarily I try to go with the flow, remain impassive and nonjudgmental, when families behave strangely, but there were decisions that we had to make that night. I asked why this news made them happy.

The son answered my question in measured words. "You are the first one," he said, "who thinks that my father will survive."

The snow had stopped. Plows and sanders had done their jobs; the drive home was easy. The next morning I made the arrangements to transfer Mr. Steiner to our hospital. I needed a special rocking bed to maintain his blood pressure and to prevent bedsores, and special duty nurses around the clock. I needed a bed on a hospital floor staffed to handle a quadriplegic patient. I had to verify the availability of these things.

His recovery took a very long time. My predictions mostly came true. He developed pneumonia and recovered, then heart failure and recovered, and other complications and recovered. We started physical therapy, for the chest and for the arms and legs and joints, even for the eye that had turned askew. After some months, when he seemed stable, we sent him back to the first hospital, nearer to his home, with full-time nurses, and with my promise that I would stop in on weekends when I was nearby.

A little more than a week later he complained of stomach pain. The doctors found that his intestine had burst. That complication can be lethal within hours, but, his doctors told me by telephone, he had been like this for a couple of days and still looked good. I was not reassured. The medications he was taking could easily hide a serious infection. We sent an ambulance to bring him back to our hospital. I called in a surgeon whom I trusted.

The standard treatment for this complication is immediate surgery. This time, because the surgeon doubted that Mr. Steiner would survive, we tried to find the damaged part of the intestine—from the outside. Our examinations pointed to a hole low in the intestinal tract, most likely a bubble on the intestinal wall. Reviewing the records, we estimated that it had occurred about a week before. It was therefore likely that scar tissue had begun to cover the hole. That was good luck. The body's attempt at healing would eventually fail, but we knew that the temporary healing would hold for at least several more days. The surgeon suggested treating with antibiotics first, until Mr. Steiner was more stable, then later operating to make the repair. I was skeptical. We argued; he convinced me that his plan was better than mine. His decision turned out to have been good. Mr. Steiner slowly grew stronger. The operations came later. First a colostomy, done under local anesthesia. When his strength improved more the surgeon did a formal repair. When Mr. Steiner recovered from all that we sent him to a rehabilitation hospital, then, many months later, to his home.

I made weekend house calls as I had promised. His local doctor took care of Mr. Steiner's immediate needs. The stress of the illness and of the now long confinement took their toll. Mrs. Steiner, who had been unshakable during the critical period, grew edgy and tense. Mr. Steiner himself became depressed. Mrs. Steiner began to work outside the home, and the tension eased.

One day Mr. Steiner pointed out to me that a bit of motion had come to his left hand, and that the little motion he already had in his right hand had increased. Then movement, in small increments, came back to other parts. In his wheelchair, he was able to go to a therapeutic pool near his home. Assisted exercise in the pool became unassisted swimming. He set himself goals: so many laps by such and such a date. His endurance and his strength increased. Soon he was able to swim a mile a day, then two, then three, using his arms alone (his legs had not yet recovered).

He began to come to my office in his wheelchair, while physical therapy continued at home. He started to work at his job from his home. He was fortunate. He had good disability insurance and sympathy from his firm. He remained on their rolls during his extended illness. Most others would have lost their jobs. Later he went by wheelchair to his office.

As he improved, his visits to my office became less frequent and mine to his home ceased. In my office, examining him was tedious because it was difficult to move him from his wheelchair to the examining bed. It took two people to get him up and down.

Once, when I left to find an aide to help, he said, "Excuse me, I want to show you something."

His wife took forearm crutches from under her long winter coat and handed them over to him. He fitted the crutches to his arms, and then, without a word, he rose and walked out of the room.

The three of them, Mr. and Mrs. Steiner and his private nurse, waited outside the examining-room door, grinning ecstatically, grins I understood this time, when I regained my composure and raced out to verify that what I had just seen was true.

Specialists. Experience. Judgment calls. They do make differences. How often they change the course of one patient's illness is hard to say. One in ten? One in one hundred? One in one thousand? I have never counted. I don't think anyone has or can.

It would be nice to believe that any doctor in any small hospital would and could always make the right decision, rarely need a consultation, or an exotic consultation for a rare disease, but that is not true. Experience is important. Judgments differ among doctors, and sometimes calling in an expert helps. It is best when this happens by easy communication—calling an old classmate, arguing the pros and cons of different treatments with a surgeon you know well, or the like. Extreme formality, on the other hand—doctors asking insurers for permission to consult, arguing to reverse when that permission is denied—encumbers the process beyond measure. It was important that Mr. Steiner's doctor knew my colleague's very special skills. It was important that my colleague knew my lesser but adequate talent and the personal circumstances that made the distant consultation easy for me to do.

Informal channels are a powerful force for the good. Referral networks in which doctors truly feel comfortable take years to build. It saddens me to think that people unconnected with a patient's problem, connected to a patient only by the cash nexus, can and do now prohibit such referrals. Special expertise and special relationships have value. In this new era of medical care, when we destroy these informal links, how much will we lose?

ER

I watch *E.R.* on Thursday nights. This popular television drama is very self-assured. *E.R.*'s patients have simple lives and single moods. Illness comes quickly and recedes the same way, or the patients die. On *E.R.* diagnoses are quick and sure. Some of the patients are complainers—their anxieties are meant to amuse. Other patients are unrealistically hopeful, pressured, or calm. Once introduced into the show, they have temperaments that seldom change. Their medical needs have this sequence: one complaint, one diagnosis, one treatment leads (most times) to one cure.

Before my beeper stopped chirping, I picked up a phone. I was in the middle of being on rounds in my hospital.

"I have this lady in my office," my colleague said. "Can you get to her soon? Her joints are very swollen, and she is in a lot of pain. It's sort of an emergency."

"Okay." I paused, running different scenarios before my eyes. "ER? Or will my office do?" I hadn't planned to be in my office that day. But the ER was not necessarily the best place. Triage is the ER rule. In the ER, coronaries trump arthritis and hemorrhage outweighs pain. Arthritis as an ER complaint ranks low. Because a doctor is always on call in the ER, the lady might be seen at once, or, if the ER is busy, four hours from now. The ER doctor would start an evaluation, perhaps begin emergency treatment, or defer all decisions until I came.

"Better in your office," my colleague replied, of the same mind as I. "Please squeeze her in soon." I called my secretary to alert her to the change in our day. She already knew. She had screened and forwarded my colleague's call, and she had guessed what I would say.

An hour later, now in my lab, I heard my beeper chirping again. "You'd better come down right away," my secretary said. "The poor girl looks very sick. I already put her into an examining room."

As I entered the room, Marcie Ginsburg Calabrese winced with obvious agony. Her face colorless, her black hair accenting the pallor, she wore a nightgown in midday—witness to her pain. Her mother gently stroked her daughter's arm. Her brother stood grimly by.

Mrs. Calabrese anxiously watched to see where I would place my hands, watchful lest I hurt her more. To look at her was to know torment. A Kollwitz sketch in anomalous colors, elbows flexed, hands bloated like foam-rubber balls, hips and knees at right angles, knees and ankles twice their normal size, she lay rigid and immobile except for her eyes. I saw why she had not changed her clothes—for how many days? The sleeves of her nightgown could not pass over her swollen hands. I lightly touched her wrist. The joint was hot. For the moment, this information was enough. Why waste any more time?

"Private room (if we have one) or semiprivate?" I asked.

"Any room at all," all three answered at once.

I picked up the examining-room phone and called my secretary. "Cathy, please see if you can get me an emergency/priority-one bed for this girl."

"I thought you would want one, so I already did," she replied. "Seven North, room 614, bed A."

As I left to sign the hospital's admission request papers, Mrs. Calabrese's brother came to me in the hall. "Don't worry about hospital insurance or anything like that," he said, sotto voce. "She's Manny Ginsburg's daughter. We'll take care of whatever you need."

"Manny Ginsburg?" I asked.

"Yes," he said, and paused, awaiting acknowledgment of this portentous fact.

"Who's he?" said I.

"He used to work with Vitale Padovese. Died a couple of years ago. You might have seen it in the papers," the brother explained.

Oh. Now I understood. Big-time mobs and rackets. Big enough, at least, to have earned a front-page obituary in *The New York Times*—after a natural death. I noted this news with little interest. Mafia consiglieri (or whatever) cannot protect their daughters from illness. Sickness is still the same.

The diagnosis, I thought, was unambiguous. We started treatment for rheumatoid arthritis that night. Within days her inflamed joints began to respond.

On *E.R.* all the needed laboratory tests come back within an hour or two. In real life the process takes more time. On *E.R.* the tests invariably confirm what the doctors suspect. In real life doctors are often surprised by the answers, and I was this time. Mrs. Calabrese's tests for rheumatoid arthritis came back normal, telling me my first guess was wrong. Tests for lupus were, however, unexpectedly positive. I reexamined her. Despite the blood tests, she still looked as if she had rheumatoid arthritis, right down to the telltale little bumps on her elbows. The medical residents showed her to our most senior physician. He agreed with me. Then they told him the results of her blood tests. "The tests must be wrong." He shrugged, and I felt reassured.

I chose to continue my treatment. My choice was good, for Mrs. Calabrese gradually recovered. Her blood tests changed, confirming arthritis, and the lupus tests went back to normal. She was now well. Some months later her illness recurred, this time with lupus symptoms, all the while her tests reporting arthritis this time. The disease cycled like this for a couple of years, back and forth between arthritis and lupus, with the symptoms and the laboratory tests never matching—don't ask me why. In real life, diseases do that sort of thing. Certitude occurs only on television. Real-life doctors live with doubt and carry on.

Contradiction was Mrs. Calabrese's leitmotif. Arthritis symptoms, lupus tests. Lupus symptoms, arthritis tests. Lame at times, athlete at others. When she was well she ran five miles a day. She wore a Star of David; her husband wore a cross. She had been born into Jewish Mafia, and her Italian husband's family was as honest as they come. Mrs. Calabrese's brother was an outlaw. She was not.

Mr. Calabrese needed a job, and his wife's brother found one for him in another state. "Is it legal?" she asked knowingly, needing assurance before they left. Her brother said yes, so they said their goodbyes and went. The brother's description turned out to be incomplete, for the job was a cover for an illegal drug trade. "Not in my home," Mrs. Calabrese told me when she found out. "I don't want my children to have any part of this." Within days the Calabreses came back home. They moved to a hilly, forested town deep in the northern suburbs as far away from drugs and crime as she could dream.

When well, Marcie Ginsburg Calabrese was voluble, droll, outspoken, coarse, saucy, and brazen. She was pure New York in television caricature. With hurried Brooklyn speech and instant wit, she was a real-life, unscripted Rhoda Morgenstern and Rosie O'Donnell in one. A sitcom eccentric—but with a real-life edge.

Sitcom comediennes do not fall ill. They have no passion and no dark side. Marcie Ginsburg Calabrese had another dimension. Challenge her family, or give her an order when she expected a request, and her eyes would glare, her body tense, her incessant chattering cease. Push the challenge further, her voice would drop low in pitch and power. She would tilt her head and look directly into your eyes. "You don't say that to Manny Ginsburg's daughter," she would darkly say.

That is what she must have said on that foggy morning on the school athletic track in that bucolic town where she ran each morning at the break of dawn. The young man must have angered her by thwarting her run. I imagine there would have been words. I imagine that she might have uttered her father's name. But the lioness-at-bay posture, the Mafia threat, must not have worked this one time. She was strong for her size, but he was much bigger than she. He strangled her and left her body in the woods beside the running track.

The police said he was still standing there when they came, a big, intellectually challenged man, a harmless (until then) village idiot (if I can use so politically incorrect a label) whom everybody knew. Like me, he probably had no idea who Manny Ginsburg had been, nor was he likely to have known that *E.R.* patients are supposed to have unambiguous diagnoses, one-dimensional needs, and not both light and dark sides to their lives.

2

CHOICES

BABIES

How much is a baby worth? What responsibility do taxpayers or insurance holders have to support the choices of would-be parents? Do all couples have the right to bear their own children? The very asking of these questions implies that the citizenry, or some large social unit—larger than the family—has a right to control, or at least not pay for, one's neighbor's "wise" or "unwise" reproductive decisions, and can refuse to pay for them, even.

Couples who want a baby might disagree. I have had many conversations with prospective parents, and they mostly focus not on money but on the risk of malformation, the mother's health, and chance. The discussions are intense, for we talk of very high risks. A mother's illness might worsen, she might even die, and the baby might die, too. Some of these pregnancies might seem unwise to you. Some certainly do to me. But whose value systems count when wisdom is defined?

"Please come soon," the obstetrics resident begged of me early one Friday afternoon. "She's Hasidic. She's sick, but she won't let you see her after sunset, after the Sabbath has begun."

"All right," I muttered into the telephone, rapidly restructuring my afternoon schedule, suspecting that, Sabbath or not, weekend or not, I would not leave early that night.

The patient's obstetrician had already given me a brief summary of the medical facts: she was seventeen weeks into her second pregnancy. She had a one-and-a-half-year-old daughter, Rebekkah, born prematurely of a difficult pregnancy, who had cerebral palsy. Last week her feet had swelled, then her legs, now her whole body. There was a lot of protein in her urine—a very bad sign. He drew my attention to some favorable points. Her blood pressure was normal, and the baby, as best we could tell, seemed healthy. The obstetrician had done a few blood tests already. He suspected lupus. Could I get my evaluation in before the Sabbath starts?

Forewarned, I headed to the maternity ward, skimmed her medical chart, then went to her room. As I entered, I saw that her bedside curtains were drawn. I introduced myself to the drapery, and asked permission to intrude. A male voice bade me come in.

Behind the curtains Leb and Raizl Weintraub prepared candles and tablecloths and dishes for a private Sabbath meal. Mrs. Weintraub wore her own nightgown rather than the standard, blue-flowered, open-backed hospital gown. Her billowy robe reached to the floor. Ribbons cinched ruffled hems about her wrists and neck. She wore a ritual wig so finely made that

I had to look closely to see that it was on. Normally my medical assessment begins the first moment I lay eyes on a patient, but, with Mrs. Weintraub, there was little I could see. Her eyelids and face were puffy, and the tops of her hands and feet were swollen, too. She appeared frightened.

Mr. Weintraub stood warily at her side. He wore a long black cloak. His white shirt lacked both collar and tie. A broad-brimmed hat, black slippers, a frizzled red beard, sidecurls dangling in front of his ears.

Born in America, the Weintraubs spoke to each other in Yiddish and to me in the accented, intoned, inverted-syntax English—with *th*'s and *d*'s sounding like *t*'s, broad *a*'s more like *e*'s—that reminded me of my grandparents' native tongues. I needed to examine Mrs. Weintraub, I explained. She asked me if her husband could stay. That was fine, so I pulled up a chair and began.

I have never witnessed a police interrogation, but I think it must be like the way my interview with Mrs. Weintraub began. Her eyes constantly met his to seek guidance, silently asking: May I answer that question? Taciturn, he replied with a gesture or facial expression but no words. Their glances showed mutual trust; his decisions seemed to rule. Secrecy on the part of a patient with a doctor is not so common. Initially I was puzzled, but then I sensed the dynamic of this conversation.

I took a chance. "It has to be a boy, doesn't it?" I asked. "The rebbe doesn't know about your illness, does he?"

A male child validates a marriage among Hasidic Jews. A barren woman (one who cannot produce a boy) can be divorced if the rebbe, the congregation's leader, so commands. Or the husband's parents can demand an annulment. One word from the rebbe dissolves the marriage. There is no recourse. It is God's command.

Their eyes met, paused, returned to mine, then met again.

They studied my face, I guess, and joked about the origin of my name. That connection may have helped. Mr. Weintraub nodded. The wife spoke.

"No," she answered, tears filling her eyes. "No one knows. His parents don't know. They can't know. Please."

Both Raizl and Leb Weintraub had known about her diagnosis since before Rebekkah was born, but they had told no one. They were frightened: if Raizl could not have children she would be sent away.

"Please," Raizl Weintraub now pleaded directly with me. "My husband, he's a very kind man. He understands, but his parents won't. Tell them something has happened to my kidneys because of the pregnancy, but don't tell them I knew this before." Leb Weintraub nodded assent.

What she asked us to say was mostly true. "Something" had indeed "happened" to her kidneys. Normally urine contains no protein. But when the kidneys leak more than four grams of protein a day, the amount of protein in the blood falls, and water fills the feet and legs. Raizl Weintraub's kidneys were leaking twenty-five grams per day, the most I had ever seen in a pregnant lupus patient, and the highest her obstetrician had seen in any pregnant patient. So much water had accumulated in her body that she had gained fifty pounds (all water) in just three weeks. Every part of her body was bloated. Wherever I touched her, my fingers left a dent. The protein in her blood, carrying nutrition to the baby, was dangerously low.

The obstetricians and I both doubted the baby would survive. He and I each asked the obvious question, but we knew the answer in advance: the Weintraubs would not consider an abortion. That meant we could not treat her illness in the way we would have preferred, since the best treatments would harm the baby. Second best would have to do.

The sun had not yet dipped below the horizon. I had completed my evaluation on time. I explained to the Weintraubs what I planned.

Mr. Weintraub began to instruct me about care of his wife during the Sabbath.

"Check on her frequently, because she won't be able to use the call button or any mechanical device," he said. "She can use only her Sabbath silverware. We'll bring her glatt kosher food, salt-free, whatever you want. Our community will supply what she needs."

I interrupted him. I told him she wasn't my first Hasidic patient, we knew what to do, we could get glatt kosher food, it would be okay. He laughed. "So you know about our meshugaas [craziness], do you?" Yes, we knew about their meshugaas. We began treatment before the sun went down.

Emotionally, Mrs. Weintraub's was a very long pregnancy. Of a normal pregnancy's forty weeks, she spent more than twenty on the maternity floor. Our second-best treatment worked, more or less: the protein in her urine decreased to a tolerable level and that in her blood increased to a safe level. The abnormal fluid that saturated her body went away. The baby grew. We doctors followed the Weintraubs' rules about what we said. To the parents and the rebbe we told only the half-truths that Raizl and Leb permitted us to tell. We scratched our heads, looked puzzled. "Some sort of kidney problem," we said, "but it's getting better, and the baby seems okay." I don't know if they believed us or not. To our surprise, they asked for no details. My guess is that they chose not to ask.

Mrs. Weintraub improved enough for us to give her eight-hour passes to attend religious services with her community. When the pregnancy reached thirty-seven weeks her blood pressure rose, a dangerous complication we had anticipated. High blood pressure threatens both mother and child. We decided to take no more risks. With Raizl and Leb's concurrence and with the rebbe's consent, we delivered their child by cesarean section. Moshe was small. He was healthy.

During her long hospital stay, Raizl Weintraub became comfortable with me and with the hospital staff. She often helped the nurses; she talked with and supported other frightened mothers. When we admitted another pregnant Hasidic woman to the maternity floor, she and Mrs. Weintraub became friends. But after Moshe's birth her more formal personality returned. Not sensing the change immediately, I made some social mistakes. One day, watching her rock Moshe in her arms, I said to her, "Moshe must be blessed, he must be a special child, because we hadn't expected him to survive."

A look of terror passed over her face. Only then did I remember the Yiddish expression *ka'yin ein hora*, let the evil eye stay away.* In traditional Judaism, a compliment attracts the devil, the evil eye, and puts a curse on the one being praised. Graciously understanding my ignorance, Mrs. Weintraub immediately negated my comment with a corrective prayer, recovered her composure, and smiled.

Another time she and Moshe were leaving to go home, I reached out to shake her hand. I wanted to wish her well. She jerked back, snapping her hands behind her and beyond my reach. Smiling—coquettish, if a Hasid can be a coquette—she whispered, "I'm sorry. I can't. I really can't."

Another moment of recognition for me. Though I had touched her many times at the hospital, checking for excess fluid, listening to her heart and lungs, and listening to her unborn child, it was different now. An ill Hasidic woman can

---

*I had often heard my grandmother use the expression. Since I knew little Yiddish, I thought she was saying "canine horror," although what the dog might have done at the time was a mystery to me.

be touched by her doctor. Only a husband can touch a woman who is well.

"I can't" meant "I am not a patient anymore." Walking out the door, the ritual ten paces behind her husband, her withdrawn hand said to me that she was no longer a woman with lupus but simply Raizl, wife of Leb, mother of Rebekkah, and (thank God) mother of a son.

In many ways you might call the decision Laurie and Mark Rubin made about parenthood unwise. I did when Laurie first described her plans.

At a public meeting, I had discussed lupus and pregnancy, and there was the usual question-and-answer period at the end. Afterward, almost always someone comes up to the podium with one more question, usually concerning himself.

Laurie Rubin waited quietly until all the other questioners had left, then asked for a private conversation. That wasn't a big problem, since the auditorium was now empty, but my office was nearby and more comfortable and the janitors were closing the auditorium doors. I guessed the topic of her concern. Her curly dark hair cut short, her face a little full, like someone taking cortisone, her makeup not completely hiding a telltale rash, Mrs. Rubin looked like many women I had seen before. In my office, her voice was soft, not timid, but without confidence either. She had lupus, she said. (Needlessly. I had already figured that out.) And she was a few weeks pregnant.

At my invitation, Mrs. Rubin brought her husband to my office on my next appointment day. Her mother came along. They knew that Laurie had lupus kidney disease. They had been told by other doctors that pregnancy could be dangerous for her and for the baby. The Rubins had heard of our research project on lupus pregnancies and had thought their decision through. They wanted a child. Laurie's disease seemed to be under control. They wanted to take their chances. Laurie's doctor, however, did not agree. He wanted to end the pregnancy. Would I take her as a patient? they asked. I would and I did.

Her pregnancy was difficult (an understatement). Mrs. Rubin's disease seriously worsened. Her kidneys began to fail. We gave her high doses of cortisone. Her blood pressure rose to frightening levels. Her body filled with fluid. At six months the unborn Sara stopped growing, an irregular heartbeat soon showing that she was in mortal danger. Together we—Laurie and Mark, the grandparents, the obstetrician, and I—understood: we had to deliver her immediately, very prematurely, or let her die. It was under seven months, only one and one-half pounds—the limits of the possible. The decision was unanimous. And so came Sara, like Macduff in *Macbeth*, ripped untimely from her mother's womb.

Both mother and daughter were very ill. They stayed for a long time in the hospital, Laurie for more than a month after the delivery and Sara for more than three. The bills were higher than anything I had seen before. Babies so small do not come gently into that bright day. Sara endured almost every difficulty that can complicate the life of a very premature baby. She could not eat. Her lungs were immature. She had infections. She had brain hemorrhages. She had convulsions. But she grew, survived, then thrived. Mark and the grandparents all stayed close and supportive, which was important for them all (and for me). Not all families stay together under such stress.

Was all this worth it? And if so, to whom? From the day we first talked, the Rubins knew about the catastrophes that might happen and then did happen. They had had a choice, and they chose to go ahead. They did not ask their insurance company for permission, and they did not consult taxpayers or voters. They believed that our society upholds the right of families to make such decisions, all hundreds of thousands of dollars of them.

Do you agree with the Rubins? It is easier to disagree if you don't think of Laurie and Mark and Sara as individual people, but think only abstractly: sick mother, very high-risk pregnancy, a possibly damaged baby, very high costs guaranteed. It is hard to disagree if you know the Rubins, and it is impossible to disagree when you meet Sara. Curly black hair, just like her mom, flushed cheeks, excited, cheerful, eager. Uncontained and uncontainable energy. Things are not perfect for Sara, however. She is a year behind in school, and her eyesight is a little weak, but basically she is a normal girl, loved and loving.

Her mother did not do well. Her kidneys failed when Sara was seven or eight. Sara, in school, received an assignment: write a story with pictures telling us about your mother. Here is what nine-year-old Sara wrote:

This book is about Dialysis and it is dedicated to my Mom. With love, Sara.

One day I went to dialysis with my Mom. I went to learn about dialysis. I was curious about it. My Mom goes to dialysis because her kidney doesn't work right. A kidney is an organ in your body. It helps the extra food you eat get out of our body but my Mom's kidney doesn't work. Dialysis cleans her kidney for her. She goes to Saint Mary's Hospital from 10:30 to 3:00. When she gets there the nurses weigh her and take her temperature and blood pressure. They put her on the machine and hook her up to it. The machine takes the blood out and cleans it and puts it back in. When she is on dialysis she reads, talks to the nurses, sleeps, watches TV and listens to music. When she gets off the machine the nurses take out the needles and put bandages on the marks. They weigh her again and she should weigh less because her blood has been filtered. Then she can go home. Now she is waiting to get a new kidney and when she gets one she won't have to go to dialysis anymore!!!!!!!!!!!!

THE END!

The next year life became a little easier for Laurie and Sara and Mark. Laurie received her kidney transplant and doesn't need the dialysis machine anymore. Laurie and Sara and Mark Rubin are a normal family again.

Gloria and Hector Bermudez are devout, but their piety was not on public display. It took me several years to understand. At the beginning, I did not see intense religion as a part of the life of this newly married, anxious twenty-one-year-old woman, rigid with pain and fevered because of a rare disease that inflames and distorts all the big arteries. Nor did I see it in Hector, her husband, who held two jobs to keep the family going. She and Hector asked me to make her well. They did not tell me that they were also asking God.

Mrs. Bermudez is outwardly conventional. She is modest to an unusual degree—indeed her reserve can be startling. One time, a few days after she first entered the hospital, I heard her sobbing, her bedside curtains closed. I entered and asked her what the trouble was. She told me that a group of medical students had come and, as a group, had asked her to remove her blouse so that they could listen to her heart murmur. They had not covered her breasts. Modesty is not so casually violated in the rural, Pentecostal village of her birth.

I know that students need to learn, but it was time for me to separate my physician self from my professorial self. Mrs. Bermudez, a ward patient, was not officially in my charge, but I had enough authority to require that medical students examine her only in my presence. She accepted that arrangement, in part because I was the senior physician, but more because when I examined her I let her place the stethoscope under her blouse for me. The students learned how to do this from me.

One of her heart valves leaked badly and needed repair. The surgeons replaced it with a type of valve they knew would itself have to be replaced in about ten years. (With a permanent valve, she would have had to take a dangerous medication, and pregnancy would have been precluded for the future. The surgeons had considered her age and her future in making their choice.) Though I met Mrs. Bermudez's pastor at her bedside from time to time, I did not pay him much heed. Visiting clergy are common in hospitals.

I was startled when Mrs. Bermudez returned to my clinic after her surgery. She was wearing what looked to me like a nun's white habit. Her dark hair was concealed by a white cap and scarf; her jacket, blouse, and long, simple skirt were also white. Even in health Mrs. Bermudez was very pale, and the whiteness of her garb emphasized her pallor. You saw no movement when she walked—floated, rather, like a Moiseyev dancer. Her voice was nearly inaudible. The demeanor, the clothing, the color, and the woman implied a life not quite of this world. My eyebrows lifted in wordless query. She had made a promise to God, she said, for allowing her to survive the surgery. She wore the attire for one year.

Mrs. Bermudez's health improved markedly with her new heart valve. The year of her promise passed. Now dressed normally, she brought her husband with her to a routine clinic visit. This surprised me because he still held two jobs and usually accompanied her only when she was very ill.* Shyly, looking at her feet, once again speaking just above a whisper, she told me that God had placed her on earth to produce two children; that she intended to conceive. Would I tell her and her husband the risks? I asked Mr. Bermudez if he felt the same way. Yes, he said, with apprehension, his swarthy face now ashen. He looked more like a fifteen-year-old on a first date than a man who had been married for some three years and had stood by as his wife underwent open-heart surgery. I was not very optimistic. In fact, I said, because her heart was not strong and her arteries blocked and weakened, she might die. "If God wants to take me before I have a child," she said, "that's His will, and I'll be happy." Mr. Bermudez agreed.

I worried greatly, and the obstetrician worried greatly, but Mr. and Mrs. Bermudez were secure in their faith. Her pastor, whom I noted this time, visited her regularly, in hospital and out. The pregnancy went more easily than we thought it might. A healthy child was born. Two years later, with Mrs. Bermudez's new heart valve now beginning to fail, she became pregnant again. Our conversation this time was brief. Each couple must produce two children, must replace themselves,

---

*Mrs. Bermudez had been well for some time, but one night she called me complaining of a new symptom (incoherently described—and she was usually articulate) and asked if she could see me right away. It was evening, so I arranged for her to come to the emergency room, and I alerted the residents that she was on her way. When I saw her the problem was obvious: Hector had fallen from a scaffolding at work and had been injured. He would not take time off work to seek help for himself, but he would to take her to the hospital if she were ill. She had faked new symptoms so that Hector would come to the emergency room, allowing me to see and treat him. It helped a lot that I, Hector, and the medical residents all had a sense of humor when we figured out what she had done.

she said. The rules were still the same. God would protect her once more.

Women's bodies normally add fluid during pregnancy, and the extra fluid strains the heart. Mrs. Bermudez's heart was not strong enough this second time, and the second pregnancy was difficult. She spent the last several weeks in the hospital, and when she was in the best possible condition, we delivered her second child by cesarean section. Then, when we knew the baby was healthy, at her and Hector's request, and with the consent of her pastor, we tied her Fallopian tubes. Hector and Gloria had produced two children. They had fulfilled God's commands, which is what they wanted to do. And we then replaced Mrs. Bermudez's heart valve a second time, this time with a steel-and-plastic one that would last for the rest of her life.

"I'm not gonna die?" she shouted excitedly. "I'm not gonna die?"

I wanted to bury my head in my hands and cry, or tear my hair out, or scream. But I didn't. I was tired. I answered the question. "No," I said once again in discouragement.

I had spent the last hour and a half, maybe more—it was the end of the day, I had lost track of time—telling Christina and Stavros Papadopoulos that there was absolutely no chance that she could carry a pregnancy to term, and that if she tried chances were very high that the baby would be seriously malformed. After all, her kidneys worked at only one-third of normal capacity. Despite four powerful medications, her blood pressure was hard to control, and she was taking a chemotherapy drug, cyclophosphamide, which can deform unborn children. This discussion had taken a very long time. I had explained and reexplained everything. Mrs. Papadopoulos, more fluent in English than her husband, translated each point. I don't speak Greek, but hers were not single-phrase translations. A lot passed between the two about each of my comments. Mr. Papadopoulos listened, asked questions that Mrs. Papadopoulos translated back, and on and on. Even without translation, the conversation would have been long, because my main point was not getting through. I had just given them the most negative assessment I had ever given about a patient's prospective pregnancy—impossible, can't be done, don't even try—and the only thing Mrs. Papadopoulos asked was "I can get pregnant, and I'm not gonna die?"

I don't really know what Mr. Papadopoulos heard. He asked nothing more, and I could not talk directly to him. I did learn that it was not religion that drove their decision. They wanted a baby for themselves.

"No," I said, "I don't think you're going to die, but there will be no baby. You may get very sick. Yes, we'll take care of you, whatever you decide."

Three months later she came back cheerful, even giddy. She was pregnant. She had stopped taking cyclophosphamide on her own.

Her blood pressure was much too high, but her kidneys maintained their borderline function. We juggled her medications, added this, took away that, but we knew that it was futile. At twelve weeks the baby stopped growing. At sixteen weeks the baby died. The pregnancy was over. No, she did not die, but the baby, as we knew it would, did.

If your only criterion of value is how much money (in taxes or in insurance premiums) it will cost when one couple and their doctor undertake an "unwise" pregnancy, you might disagree with the Weintraub, Rubin, Bermudez, or Papadopoulos families. They, after all, decided to spend tens of thousands of dollars, mostly of other people's money. Did they have the right to do that? Should we say no to the Rubins or Weintraubs, the Bermudezes or Papadopouloses, because their decisions are not cost-effective? The problem is that it is wrong to use only the cost criterion to answer the question. Other legitimate values are at play. Raizl Weintraub and Laurie Rubin were already pregnant when the question was raised. Mrs. Rubin's other doctor had told her she needed an abortion. I suggested one to Mrs. Weintraub, but the Weintraubs' faith prohibited ending a pregnancy this way. Of the four couples, only the Rubins could have (with repugnance) chosen abortion—had they believed that either Laurie or Sara would die—but doctors disagreed about the risk to both. Faced with uncertainty, they could not terminate the pregnancy. Others, given the same odds, might have chosen differently.

I am not opposed to abortion, nor is the obstetrician with whom I worked. We have both advised women facing worse odds to end their pregnancies. In fact, that is what we told the Papadopouloses. We both thought that the Rubins' decision was risky but not impossible, and we so advised. We said the same to the Weintraubs and Bermudezes. But parents, informed of the risks, are the ones who make the choice in the end. Doctors support their choice and make the best of it. Personal values, not societal values, rule. Faith counts. In the long run, as public policy, this counts more than the dollar cost of high-risk pregnancies.

Expensive illnesses occur by chance, usually, and we accept, or used to accept, society's responsibility to support the patients who are their victims. But if an expensive illness occurs by choice—and in many minds, the pregnancy of an ill woman is certainly a choice—is society still obliged? One answer is that if we respect religion, we must also respect the choices people make based on religion, whatever the cost. For those with deep religious beliefs, pregnancy is not a choice; reproduction is a gift from and an obligation to God, they would and did say. We cannot superimpose different beliefs on these couples and say, "You did not have to get pregnant, and we won't pay." We also cannot say, "It is okay for you, Raizl and Leb Weintraub, Laurie and Mark Rubin, Gloria and Hector Bermudez, to go ahead with your pregnancies, because you believe in God," and then refuse to support the pregnancies of others because they believe in a different God or in no God at all.

The question is open to debate whether we are obliged to pay for costly medical care when religion is a proximate cause for its need. The debate will show that religion contributes to the policy, but if we deny the religious basis of medical choice, then we deny one of the foundations of our nation. Do we then have the right to reject a choice—like the Papadopouloses'—that has no religious basis? The answer of course is no. Choices are equal, whether or not we (doctors? taxpayers? moralists?) agree with them.

To exclude pregnancy costs from insurance coverage is to impose the cost of an elected health need on the chooser. Do we really want to do that? The important point is to know that the exclusion is a kind of rationing, and to ask whether pregnancy should be rationed.

WASTED DOLLARS?

Nick d'Abruzzi is the only patient I ever fired. After being his doctor for five years, I told him I would not see him again. I asked for and got the equivalent of a restraining order that kept him from consulting me, and I removed myself from all responsibility concerning his care.

In the beginning I was more accepting of Mr. d'Abruzzi. I had become his doctor when his own physician moved to another state, at which point I had known him for about five years. He was a "character" in our hospital. I had seen him with my colleague from time to time during his periodic hospital admissions and clinic visits.

Mr. d'Abruzzi's image of himself differed from mine of him. I thought of him as an argumentative man of low intelligence whose life and future had been seriously damaged by a disfiguring disease. He thought of himself as a pint-sized Sylvester Stallone. He wanted to be powerful and threatening, but as I saw it, he was a neighborhood joke. At least it seemed that way the several times each year when he came to the hospital to be patched up following a barroom brawl that had not ended in his favor. Illness had made the skin on Mr. d'Abruzzi's hands so tight and scarred that he could neither open nor close his fingers nor make a good fist, a reason he lost the barroom fights.

Despite his bodybuilding efforts, tough-guy street speech, and anger, Mr. d'Abruzzi was an unlikely Sylvester Stallone. For one thing, he was small, maybe five feet six, less than one hundred thirty pounds. For another, his illness, scleroderma, and his drug addiction handicapped him greatly. Scleroderma (*sclero* means scarred and *derma* means skin) is a rare disease that tightens and hardens the skin and sometimes damages internal organs as well. Most patients with scleroderma have episodes of blood-vessel spasm: the circulation to fingers or toes suddenly shuts off, making them painful or numb, and then opens again. The individual fingers turn red, white, or blue, off and on, like blinking bulbs on an American flag marquee. Anxiety makes this happen, and cold does, too. Mr. d'Abruzzi had had a severe blood-vessel spasm, as a result of which he had lost the tips of most of his fingers. They had blackened, shriveled, and fallen off, in a process doctors call autoamputation. You can imagine how horrible it looks. Autoamputation today frightens those who see it much as leprosy used to frighten others in ancient times. Strangers shun persons with scleroderma for this reason and for other plainly visible skin changes. There is not much good you can say about the disease. But for Mr. d'Abruzzi, when he was arrested by the police, which was often, mostly for disturbing the peace, it sometimes helped: the police officers usually looked at his hands and let him go.

In scleroderma patients, a spasm in the blood vessels can happen in the sex organ, which causes impotence. Mr. d'Abruzzi was impotent at least some of the time. His sexual desire, he insisted (often), was normal, even more than normal, he would say. Impotence was one of the reasons for his anger, and also for his addiction.

Mr. d'Abruzzi did not have many women friends. Mostly he purchased sex from women vendors on the street. When he was not impotent he was usually unlucky. Periodically I treated him for venereal disease. Other times his attempts at sex failed. If the hired lady was impolite enough to laugh, he usually beat her up. (He told me this was the only appropriate response.) But then her pimp would beat him up, and he would come back to the emergency room for patching once again.

Mr. d'Abruzzi believed that his sexual performance improved when he took large amounts of Tuinal, a type of sleeping pill then popular among drug users, and Valium, a tranquilizer. I opined that those drugs impeded his sexual power, but he disagreed. I had not introduced him to those medicines, but I prescribed them because I could not merely withdraw them without causing him harm. I also prescribed them to keep the peace. He argued, vehemently, with me to keep the prescriptions coming. The prescriptions were a source of conflict between us. I would provide one month's supply; he would return in a week or so with an unconvincing excuse to have the prescription refilled: "I lost the pills in the subway," or "I was robbed," or "My mother flushed them down the toilet." I assumed that he sold the extra pills. After a while I set a rule: only one prescription each month, regardless of what might happen. Then I learned that another physician, in another hospital, had been giving him duplicate prescriptions, from before the time I had assumed his care. With Mr. d'Abruzzi's knowledge, I spoke to the other physician. We agreed that I would prescribe no more drugs. The other physician was unwilling to stop.

To deal with the behavior and the drugs, I sent Mr. d'Abruzzi to psychiatrists and to a drug addiction program, to no avail. The psychiatrists said he had a low tolerance for frustration. Borderline intelligence made the problem nearly insoluble. This was a dilemma, because Mr. d'Abruzzi had a lot to be frustrated about. When he was angry, he turned very blue, and he trembled and screamed. It was all rather unnerving if you did not know him. Angry, blue, and trembling, he often roamed the hospital to find me in my laboratory, my private office, or on the hospital floors. He frightened my secretary, my laboratory technician, and other people on our staff.

Mr. d'Abruzzi was the reason I unlisted my home telephone number. When he was disgruntled about something, which was often, he would call me at ten-minute intervals throughout the night. At each call he'd ask the same questions, never something I could answer easily. I canceled my listed telephone number, unlisted the new one, and made him call my answering service instead. At long intervals—once or twice a night—the service gave me the count of his calls. The operators were very unhappy with me and with him, but over time he called less often.

Because of his tight skin and poor circulation, Mr. d'Abruzzi from time to time developed open sores on his hands and feet. One winter he developed a painful sore on one of his toes, which I tried to treat in the outpatient department. I cleaned it, bandaged it, and gave him new medications to improve his circulation. I asked him to stay off his feet and to keep his foot very warm and dry, a conservative approach which works for most people. For the first week or two he did not improve. A week after that, driving through Mr. d'Abruzzi's neighborhood, I stopped for a traffic light. There, on the corner, standing in a snowbank, wearing light (not waterproof) sneakers, stood Mr. d'Abruzzi, very high, intoxicated, on what I did not know. At least whatever he had swallowed or injected or smoked did not smell like alcohol or marijuana. I know how he smelled because he saw me waiting for the light, staggered to my car, and in what I assume he thought was Stallone-like gallantry leaned into the window, which I opened, and incoherently introduced himself to my wife and five-year-old daughter. He held up traffic through the next light change, then lurched back to the snowbank and sat down. I understood that the ulcer was unlikely to heal.

The reason I fired Mr. d'Abruzzi was that I became frightened for my family. The snowbank was the beginning. At his next clinic visit I told Mr. d'Abruzzi that I would admit him to the hospital as soon as there was an available bed. We had three priority ranks for admissions: emergent (a patient in immediate danger of deterioration or death; the hospital would put an extra bed in the hallway if necessary); urgent (likely to deteriorate in days, patient will get the next available bed);

and elective (anything else). Even though a three-week-old foot ulcer merits only elective priority, I assigned Mr. d'Abruzzi to the urgent list. A bed would be available within a day or two. This solution did not satisfy Mr. d'Abruzzi, who went directly to the admitting office himself. They confirmed the news. He called the admitting resident. He said the same.

Mr. d'Abruzzi found our response unacceptable. He went home, picked up a baseball bat, returned, and (blue, trembling, and screaming) demanded immediate admission. A hospital security guard tried to stop him. Mr. d'Abruzzi swung, hit his target, and broke the guard's arm. The guard called the police. The police arrested Mr. d'Abruzzi. The hospital's chief administrator then called me in a panic. He envisioned headlines in the tabloids: "Hospital Sends Sick Patient to Jail." The administrator went down to the precinct headquarters, posted bond, and brought him back to the hospital for admission, in handcuffs, a police guard in tow. Then he paid the hospital guard to drop the assault charges. Mr. d'Abruzzi was released from custody, the handcuffs were removed, and the police officer was allowed to leave. Mr. d'Abruzzi had gotten what he wanted, a bed in the hospital, albeit in the visitors' lounge at the end of the hall, because there truly had been no available beds.

A few months later Mr. d'Abruzzi, frustrated about something else and knowing the route I took when I walked my daughter to kindergarten each day, reminded me of his baseball bat and threatened me: "I'll get you," he said, "and I'll get your daughter, and I'll get anyone who tries to stop me"— if I didn't do whatever he wanted that day.

I went to the hospital administrators, who referred me to the police. The police told me that threats to me did not merit protective action. (The assault on the guard, they thought, did not predict future assaults on me or on my daughter.) They said they would come immediately if he actually tried to attack me or my daughter. This was not reassuring. I went back to the hospital administrators and asked them to declare Mr. d'Abruzzi persona non grata at our hospital. The administrators and their lawyers demurred, but we eventually negotiated a compromise. Mr. d'Abruzzi would be restricted to the hospital's clinic, pharmacy, and blood-drawing areas. He would no longer have an assigned physician (no one else would accept him), but only whichever doctor was on call. He would receive no prescriptions except those directly related to scleroderma. He had to attend psychiatric counseling sessions. He was to have no contact with me again. Any violations of the restrictions and he would be officially persona non grata at our hospital. We would assist in a transfer of his care.

Mr. d'Abruzzi did not want to go to another hospital. He obeyed our rules, and things stayed quiet for a couple of years, until he was arrested again for something that involved carrying or using or firing a gun (I don't know the details)—which must have been difficult because of his damaged fingers—and he was convicted and sent to an upstate prison, where he later died, I am told, before the age of thirty, of a complication of scleroderma.

"One of your lupus patients came in pretty sick last night, but we buffed her up and she's okay now," the emergency-room resident, overly smug, told me early one morning. The resident was one I liked, eager, like all good doctors, to make a better diagnosis or carry out a more brilliant therapeutic maneuver, to show his teachers how good he was. Nonetheless I was concerned that I had not been called. I asked for details. The patient had come in about two in the morning, he said. She had begged him not to wake me up. He had assessed her complaint—a straightforward problem, he thought—had begun treatment, and had sent her directly to the hospital floor. I could find her on Payson 4.

He had had a busy night. Shuffling through papers to find his notes, he did not fully recall her name. "Susan something," he guessed. He drew a verbal portrait: white, mid-twenties, about five feet two, dark hair, overweight, complaining of chest pain, good story for pulmonary embolus (which she had had before), blood-clotting studies a little funny. She had responded to treatment quickly and was now stable.

I had been listening uneasily, but now I laughed out loud. Guffawed would be a better word. It was a "gotcha" moment.

"That has to be Susan Sandman," I told him, one-upping him this time. "You didn't look at the front-desk picture file. You admitted someone with Munchausen's syndrome. She needed no treatment at all."

In the late eighteenth century, Baron Karl Friedrich Hieronymus von Münchhausen told outrageous tales of his prowess in battle. Rudolf Erich Raspe published the tales, and they are told to this day; they were the topic of a popular movie in 1989. At some time long ago, I'm not sure when, Baron Münchhausen's name entered medical lore. (The English spelling of the name is a corruption.) This is not just a little moaning or limping now and then, but major untruths: Munchausen patients cough or vomit blood, induce fever, and inject themselves with infectious material to produce abscesses. Munchausen's syndrome patients subject themselves to every medical assault a doctor can make upon them. They beg for tubes to be inserted, they undergo repeated surgeries, and they accept treatments with toxic medications in order to fulfill their deep, and poorly understood, psychiatric needs. They are very convincing patients. They wouldn't be Munchausen patients if they were not.

Like most patients with factitious illness, Susan Sandman
had started her career with doctors with a genuine medical
problem in her past. Evaluating her as a teenager for a non-
descript problem, a doctor had noted an abnormal blood-
clotting test, slightly suggestive, but only suggestive, of lupus.
Her doctor went no further to confirm his suspected diagnosis,
assuming that the blood test explained her symptoms, and
began treatment with very powerful medications. He died a
short while later. She went to other doctors. They said the first
doctor was wrong. But Ms. Sandman had learned that some
of her complaints attracted their attention, and had learned
that a suspected complication, a blood clot in the lung, could
not be immediately disproved. When she appeared in an emergency room complaining of the right symptoms, she usually
gained admission, no questions asked.

Ms. Sandman knew I was unconvinced that she had lupus.
At her first admission to our hospital, she offered me additional proof: she had once had, she said, the characteristic
"butterfly" rash. But I had not seen her with that rash, I replied. When I made rounds the next day her cheeks were flam-
ingly red. "The rash came out," she said, hopefully. I liked the
attempt. A lupus rash typically has sharp borders; her rash
faded at the edge. (The nurse later told me that she had seen
Ms. Sandman vigorously rubbing her face with the coarse hem
of her bedsheets to make her face turn red.) See, she seemed
to say, her eyes questioning, a bit desperate, when I entered
her room. Doesn't this prove I have lupus? I told Ms. Sandman
that her new rash was an important clue. Adding that I wanted
to document the rash for the medical record, I sent her to the
medical photography laboratory for a picture. She was very
pleased. It is a nice picture. It shows a happy young woman,
head tilted slightly to the right, a little seductive, eyes spar-
kling, looking directly into the lens, with a charming smile.

I had lied. I made copies of the picture. I posted one in our emergency room in the file that emergency rooms keep of patients who under false pretenses seek admission or drugs and whom the hospital prefers to keep out. I then asked the medical students assigned to her case to take other copies to all the emergency rooms in New York to see how many admissions they could find. The students documented seventeen admissions in four hospitals under six different names within approximately two years. This was an interesting problem, so we presented her story as a teaching case at medical grand rounds. Several hundred doctors were present. A member of the audience, visiting from a hospital across town, spoke from the floor: he knew her, too. So it was eighteen admissions and five hospitals. (I have no idea how she paid for these admissions. Probably the hospital had checked no records and found too late that the name she used had been false.) I suspect that I violated some privacy regulations in sending her picture around, but personal privacy was not a big issue in those days.

Armed with the medical students' documentation, late in the day I went to Ms. Sandman's room. Most Munchausen syndrome patients abruptly flee when confronted, but I had sought advice from our psychiatrists earlier. I went alone and closed the door. I sat on the edge of her bed so we could talk. We had known each other for a while, so she listened quietly to what I had to say. I told her what I had done with the picture, why, and what we had found. I apologized for my dishonesty. I told her we could work together to help her get over this problem. I would still be her doctor and would talk to her when she was frightened. I would be open-minded if she developed new symptoms, so long as she did not tell other doctors that she had lupus. I would not admit her to the hospital unless I felt there was real proof of need. She did not flee. I discharged her from the hospital the next morning. She came to my clinic the next week. She enrolled in a psychiatric treatment program, keeping an appointment we had arranged before she had gone home.

Over the next few years things worked well. She came to my clinic every month or two. We sometimes talked on the telephone between visits. Two or three times another hospital called me to tell me they had admitted her and that she had asked them to call me to explain her illness to them. Not perfect, but an improvement. Then there was the admission the resident misdiagnosed; then there were no more hospital admissions at all.

Susan Sandman married. We three, Ms. Sandman, her fiancé, and I, had a long conversation before the wedding. Her fiancé himself had had some medical problems; each understood the other's needs. Years later she developed asthma. A doctor friend of mine who was expert in that disease gradually took over her care, and, except for his periodic comments to me, I lost contact with Ms. Sandman.

But that was long after I had personally taken the "Munchausen syndrome" label from her hospital chart and her picture from the emergency-room book.

Early on the first Wednesday of every month except August, never mind the weather, Lettie Chebowicz was the first to arrive for the 9 a.m. arthritis clinic. She sat in the waiting-area chair nearest my room. (In August she went to a camp for the elderly in the Catskill Mountains. She came for an extra visit in late July to prepare.) Eager to be first, she arrived well before check-in, sometimes before the clinic doors opened. When that happened she waited patiently in the hospital lobby. She never went to the cafeteria for coffee; it would have worried her too much to lose her place in line. To get to the clinic she came from her apartment in the Bronx, taking four different buses. Her trip took at least an hour and a half. I shuddered when I thought of her preparations. Considering the trip, the visit, the wait to have blood drawn, another wait at the pharmacy, then the return home, she put in a full day for a fifteen-minute examination. She was not a young woman. In fact, she was in her eighties. I offered, but she declined, transfer of her care to clinics nearer her home.

Lettie Chebowicz was a prototype grandmother, but she was not a grandmother. About five feet tall, maybe less, very round, chucklingly cheerful most of the time, she seemed to enjoy her clinic visits. I understood that Mrs. Chebowicz had been a widow for a very long time. She spoke little of the past. I knew that she had come from somewhere in Central Europe, Czechoslovakia, I thought. On rare occasions she would speak tenderly of her childhood in a small rural town and of a sister who had died. She once showed me a picture of this sister, standing alone, on a muddy farm, in some unidentifiable place. At other times she spoke about her daughter, her only child, who lived in California, and who, she said, suffered from mental illness. She never spoke of her husband. I think that Mrs. Chebowicz had come to New York before the Holocaust. There were no tattooed numbers on her arm.

She looked Central European. She wore wool skirts that nearly touched her ankles, mostly in muted plaids or pepper-and-salt weaves, always brown or gray, and heavy shoes. Her wool cardigan sweater never matched the skirt. She wore thick eyeglasses, with the earpieces attached to the bottoms of the eyepieces European style. She covered her hair with a babushka. In rain, she covered the babushka with plastic.

Every Christmas season, despite my protests, Mrs. Chebowicz gave me a holiday card. "Gave" is probably not the right word. Wordlessly, she stuck an envelope with my name on it in the large pocket of my white coat as she walked out the door. There was always a gracious note and a five-dollar bill folded within. I hated that. It felt as if she was giving me a tip to treat her. The cost of her care was billed by the clinic to Medicare. Clinic doctors are paid salaries, and are not paid directly by the patients. But she saw it as expressing appreciation, I knew, and I hope I was courteous in my thanks.

Mrs. Chebowicz did not have a life-threatening or crippling disease. Her knees had bowed a bit and hurt—osteoarthritis—which is why she came to the clinic. Sometimes her back bothered her, and sometimes pains went down her legs. She used a cane. Tylenol helped, and she took nothing more. She worried about diabetes, which she did not have. She demanded that I test her blood sugar at every visit. Occasionally the result showed a level that was too high. I would express concern. "I noshed a little bit," she would say. We discussed the trade-off for lowering the sugar: "Nosh to your heart's content, and soon you'll need pills, or maybe insulin shots," I would tell her. She would promise to nosh less and she would, for a while, and her sugar would come down, then the cycle would start over again. Her blood pressure was mostly normal—I had to begin each visit by measuring it—except one day it was very high. I asked if there might be an explanation. "I had a little trouble," she told me. "I was mugged coming to clinic." She was not hurt. Her purse never carried anything she could not afford to lose. A mugging was not important enough to interfere with her appointment.

For most of the time that I knew her, I don't think I recommended anything for Mrs. Chebowicz that actually required a prescription. She filled her medical requirements at the clinic pharmacy, which needed a written order even for over-the-counter medications like aspirin and acetaminophen. By my accounting, her visits were social. Even the monthly test of her blood sugar was a social act. From time to time I suggested that she might come in three months, or six months, for her next appointment. She always said no. She would see me again the first Wednesday of next month.

In winter, Mrs. Chebowicz wore many layers of clothing. I knew this because my listening to her heart every visit was another ritual, and it took a lot of time to get my stethoscope to the right layer. I was not certain that she could dress herself unassisted or that she had heat in her apartment, because my eyes and my nose told me she did not bathe often when the weather was cold. I worried about her shopping and about her ability to prepare meals. Our social service department checked her home and thought things were satisfactory. Her daughter did not visit, she complained, was selfish and did not worry about her mother. But then, Mrs. Chebowicz continued, her daughter was mentally ill. I sympathized and absorbed, by osmosis, annoyance with the absent daughter. I saw before me an elderly woman who needed the help that a daughter could give.

During one visit, Mrs. Chebowicz seemed distraught. "My daughter, she's so sick," she said. Her daughter had just undergone a mastectomy, I learned, and Mrs. Chebowicz could not afford to go to California to give care. "She's not so young, either," said Mrs. Chebowicz of the daughter. "She's sixty-five." I blinked. For some reason that does not speak well of how my mind works, I had imagined the daughter to be thirty or forty years old, and rich. She was neither.

Mrs. Chebowicz developed a chest pain when she walked, which indicated that her coronary arteries had become blocked. I gave her nitroglycerin tablets but the chest pains continued to come. I sent her to the cardiology clinic. The cardiologists tried different medicines with incomplete success. She was not a candidate for bypass surgery, the cardiologist said.

One day another short, round lady accompanied Mrs. Chebowicz to the clinic. The resemblance, except for the American manner and dress of the second lady, made it obvious that this was her daughter, who appeared to be a fully competent woman with no hint of mental illness, and appropriately concerned.

The younger woman asked to talk to me in private. "I want to take my mother home with me," the daughter said. "I've put an extra room in my house." There were tears in Mrs. Chebowicz's eyes at this proposal. She had lived decades in her apartment in the Bronx. Her husband's things were still there, she said—the first that I had heard her mention him. She did not want to go, but she agreed to try it for a month. I gave her prescriptions for three months, just in case, and a written medical summary. Her daughter knew doctors in the event an emergency occurred. As I guessed it would, the one month became two and then three. Mrs. Chebowicz returned to New York for a few more months, then moved permanently to California. She sent me cards (no five-dollar bills) for a while. Then the cards stopped coming.

All doctors know patients who waste resources. But most of the patients would not consider their behavior wasteful. Patients who seem to waste resources (as health economists count) are asking for reassurance and for someone to care about them. Some are lonely, and they come to doctors to have someone to talk to. They medicalize a social need. To call it a doctor's visit and not a paid chat gives their need validity.

In pre-cellular phone days, when I was on call on Saturday nights, as I was driving home my beeper would often sound. I'd have to stop, find a telephone, call the answering service, take the message, call the caller back, only to hear, "I'm at the drugstore. It closes in a few minutes. I thought I would refill my prescription. Will you speak to the pharmacist, please?" I used to get very angry about these calls. My mood was not improved by heavy rain if I was shoving quarters into a telephone in an uncovered roadside booth. It is so much easier and safer to fill prescriptions from the office, I would whine silently to myself, when the medical chart is available, and I can recheck doses and allergies and contraindications. Why at nine on a Saturday night? After many such calls I finally understood. These calls were not about refilling prescriptions. They were about this: "Does anyone care that I'm alive?"

Unnecessary doctor's visits are mostly asked for by patients, not by doctors. Mrs. Chebowicz, if I dared suggest a three- or six-month return, would immediately protest. "Can't I come sooner?" she would say. Mr. d'Abruzzi and Ms. Sandman assumed that any service was theirs for the asking. Patients like Mrs. Chebowicz manipulate the medical-care system in a pathetic way, and it makes one sad. Patients like Mr. d'Abruzzi and Ms. Sandman manipulate the system in an exasperating, narcissistic way. Both types are well known to doctors. Look up the topic "hateful patient" in medical journals: there are many types described. The articles tell doctors how to prevent anger from clouding their judgment and how to use psychology to get the patient to do what the doctor thinks is best. Mastering these techniques is medicine's art. What I did when I told Ms. Sandman that I thought she had Munchausen's syndrome was deliberate, not artifice, but the style is the result of training.

What the medical-journal articles do not teach us is how doctors caring for wasteful patients should protect the nation's fiscal health. Simply turn them away? Some doctors might have found it easier than did I to tell a Mr. d'Abruzzi or a Ms. Sandman that the complaints were not worthy of attention or would be treated only if the patient followed the rules. Some doctors, I know, can tell a Lettie Chebowicz to come back only when she is "really" ill. But I cannot. Inhumanity and callousness aside, even Munchausen's patients do die of something. Ms. Sandman did develop asthma, and Mr. d'Abruzzi did die, probably of scleroderma. I assume that Mrs. Chebowicz died of her coronary disease.

I suspect, as we ration health-care more, that the Susan Sandmans, the Nick d'Abruzzis, and the Lettie Chebowiczes of this world will simply be ousted from the hospitals, be turned into medical derelicts, or be assigned to less expensive professionals—a social worker perhaps. Perhaps that will be good. Dependency, mental deficiency, mental illness, and loneliness—none of these will be allowed to have medical care. Specific diagnoses will merit specific resources, not a penny more. I don't completely disagree with such a future. After all, I cannot truly say that the medical money spent on their care was well spent, unless understanding Susan Sandman and Nick d'Abruzzi, not as the sociopaths they surely were, and Lettie Chebowicz as the lonely woman she was, but as individuals in trouble, counts for something in medical care. Unless caring counts for something, too.

ALIENS

True heroes, my father says, are men and women like his parents. They were immigrants to the United States. Alone, poor, with five children, never having spoken a word of English, not even familiar with the Roman alphabet, they traversed a continent and an ocean to escape terror and to secure a better life for themselves and their family. Think about it and you will agree. Immigrants have a vision that is unimaginable to those of us who have grown to maturity in comfort, who have never faced significant prejudice, let alone cultural barriers, famine, pogroms, Holocaust, Cultural Revolution, Partition, or ethnic cleansing.

Those were not my first thoughts when Dr. Saeeda Jahan Hasan walked through my office door. I knew her to be a young physician, late of London, who had recently moved to the United States. She had fallen ill in England, and her London doctor, a friend of mine, had written to me several weeks before, asking me to continue her care. His letter described unstable health and serious illness. She had not yet contacted me. I told that to my friend. He located her and asked her to see me at once. She then called for an appointment. Assuming that responsibility and reliability were not her strengths, I did not look forward to our first interview.

A proud woman came in, straight of back, imperious of mien. To me, the product of small provincial American towns, she was distinctly singular. She wore a *salwaar kameez*, a silken knee-length tunic, and pantaloons embroidered with gold thread, and her pointed slippers were trimmed in gold. A translucent *dupati*, a type of shawl, encircled her neck loosely, like a necklace, with the ends draped over her shoulders to hang below her waist in back. Her jet-black hair was done up in a single long midline braid with gold threads intertwined. She could sit on her braid (she pointed out to me then and subsequently). Numerous filigree gold bracelets decorated her wrists and ankles, tinkling, announcing her stride. Hers was an entrance calculated to impress. She meant it to. I, making idle and somewhat silly conversation to put her at ease, ignorant for the nonce of the builder of the Taj Mahal, mentioned that I had another patient named Jahan. "The Jahans ruled my country," she replied, not missing a beat, and not mentioning that not all Jahans were Shahs.

My friend in London was correct about her illness. Despite an appearance of well-being, she was very ill. Antibodies were destroying her red blood cells faster than her bone marrow could make new ones. Eventually we had to take out her spleen—a drastic treatment—to protect her blood. Every year she had another complication. A heart attack, for one, a perforated appendix, and a series of other surgical problems for others. Suffice it to say that over the years I got to know Dr. Hasan and her family well.

By Pakistani standards she was well off, but money had not made her life easy. Her family was traditional. She had been married, at the age of thirteen, to an older man of her father's choice. The young woman who occasionally came with her to my office and whom she had introduced to me as her sister, turned out to be her daughter, born to her the year after her marriage. She did not tell me this at first because she thought Americans would ridicule her country's ways.

Dr. Hasan had not casually become a doctor. In her early twenties, mother and wife, she had asked permission of her husband and father to attend medical school. They had both said no. Not to be stopped, she left her husband, taking her daughter with her, and enrolled herself in medical school. When she completed her degree, she, her daughter, and her infant son went alone to London to continue her training. I never asked her why she then came to New York. Perhaps it was for job opportunities. Perhaps she anticipated less color prejudice in the United States. Perhaps she came for medical care, though the care she received in England was identical to and cheaper than that which we offered. Perhaps it was that she knew her prognosis and wanted her children to be raised on our shore. But I am guessing. It was not a topic we discussed.

Over the years, the pretense—distance, really—of our first

meeting faded. She dressed more as an American (slacks, of course; her Islamic modesty remained), yet the sense of authority, the "I'm in control" attitude, stayed. Repeatedly hospitalized for complications of her illness, she still sought, received, and performed jobs in her medical specialty, radiation oncology (X-ray therapy for cancer). From her hospital bed she studied to pass her specialist examinations, which she missed twice because she was hospitalized; I wrote explanatory letters for her and she was permitted to try again. All the while she worried about her son's grades at school—and my daughter's, too, for the children were about the same age. She worried about her daughter's future and eventual marriage in this non-Islamic land. When she visited my office she always asked first about my family, insisting on my answer before she would discuss her own health. "I'll be okay," her demeanor conveyed, "I have just a few minor inconveniences to contend with. How are you?"

A skilled observer of herself, she often substituted telephone calls for office visits. A couple of times, when she had weathered one more crisis and was recuperating at home, her frequent telephone calls ceased. Then, after a delay just short of that which would cause me to call her to check, the phone would ring and I would hear her say, with a giggle of embarrassment, "I'm in Karachi. I needed to rest." She would rush through the details in the three minutes the Pakistan telephone company allowed for overseas calls and, if necessary, call for another three minutes when her turn came around again. She would stay in Karachi for several weeks, cared for by servants and by her family, with whom she was again on good terms, occasionally calling with a progress report or asking for advice. Then she would return recovered, ready to plunge into the next phase of her life. She always brought back something from home—gold bracelets or an embroidered blouse for my daughter, a rug for my wife. I tried unsuccessfully to protest. I could refuse to accept presents for myself, she argued, but gifts for my family were for them.

Dr. Hasan never complained. When I cautioned her not to do something, she looked me in the eye, smiled, and said, the imperious tone back again, "You know I'll be all right. I can do that." Can do, even when she couldn't do.

I saw her somber only twice. As her illness progressed, she came to me, unsmiling, and declared, "I have to make my hajj."* I understood that she was thinking about her death. I didn't argue. It would not have made a difference if I had. I asked about the physical requirements of the trip. She told me about facilities for the disabled, support systems, the climate of Saudi Arabia at that time of year, and all the rest. So we worked together to make the pilgrimage possible. She made her hajj, then she went on to Karachi to rest, and then she returned to New York, studying for her specialist examinations, which she had missed once again.

The other time she was somber was the night before a scheduled heart surgery. She had a single room on a high floor of our hospital. The window faced west. I made an evening visit to discuss last-minute details. When I entered her room, the setting sun, opposite the door, blinded me as I entered. Blinking, shading my eyes, I saw Dr. Hasan in silhouette, sitting cross-legged on her bed, facing me (and the east, Mecca), in a seeming trance. Normally, she smiled when I came in. Usually she offered a pleasant greeting, even when ill or in pain. Tonight she stayed motionless, no greeting, and no acknowledgment that I was there. For a moment I was alarmed, but from the shadow her husband motioned me to stay still. The trance persisted for a minute or two. Then, in a series of

*The pilgrimage a devout Muslim makes to Mecca once in a lifetime.

rapid movements, she touched her forehead to the bed, turned her head quickly first to one side, then to the other, lips moving in prayers that I could not hear, then opened her eyes, looked at me, and smiled shyly, a little self-conscious. She looked down and whispered, "That was private. That was between me and God."

American medical residents—senior doctors, too—are often arrogant about "IMGs," international medical graduates. IMGs are not, in their minds, real doctors. American doctors tend not to dwell on what IMGs have endured, nor on the fact that IMGs are often the only doctors who will practice in the poorest sections of our American cities, as Dr. Hasan did when she was well. Dr. Hasan's special training in radiation therapy for cancer further distanced her from our residents. Radiation therapy science is far removed from that of internal medicine. The knowledge bases of the two disciplines are very different; their vocabularies are not the same. American-trained radiation therapists sometimes confuse the purposes of drugs used primarily by internists, as internists confuse the details of radiation therapy. Dr. Hasan made these types of minor errors when she discussed her illness with our medical residents. When she was ill, it was harder for her to focus on details. The residents assumed her incompetence and sneered.

One day I happened upon a resident describing Dr. Hasan to a colleague. "A crazy Pakistani," he scoffed, "who *thinks* she's a doctor." She was taking (he had written the order for) drugs that treated her disease but that impair thought processes—not a lot, and only temporarily—and other drugs that make some patients manic. Yet the resident tried to convince me that her excitement and mild confusion were her natural state. He did not consider the possibility that the drugs were a factor.

I became angry. His attitude was not only bad medicine but

arrogant and dismissive of her skills. I described to him and his colleague what I knew her life was like, and her thinking, when she was healthy. I made unflattering comparisons with him. I reminded him that what she accomplished she had accomplished alone, burdened by children, and threatened and periodically laid low by a potentially lethal disease. I don't think I impressed him—in fact, I assume he thought I was a pompous fool.

Dr. Hasan was aware, as I suspect most IMGs were, of what some of our homegrown doctors thought of her, but she had an inner sense of self-worth that allowed her to transcend the pettiness. That evening the residents, now annoyed at me for my outburst, came back to tell me they had proof that she was surely crazy. First, she had run out of her room, dragging her IV pole behind her, screaming that men were coming through the wall. Now, they said, she was running around, making ridiculous faces, and telling people her tongue was stuck to the roof of her mouth. They hadn't checked why she had said either of those things.

I did. There were indeed men coming through the wall: a construction crew working in another section of the hospital had done something on her floor, drilling too deeply in the wrong direction and into her room. And she was, indeed, making uncontrolled contortions of her face. Had the residents tried to understand her garbled speech, they would have heard her tell them that she was suffering an important (and, fortunately, easily reversible) side effect of the antinausea drug they had prescribed, an obvious diagnosis they should have made.

I do not know whether our residents were humbled or not. I do not know that they could be humbled. But when this crisis had passed and when she felt well again, Dr. Hasan laughed at their arrogance. This young lady, who had crossed

a continent and an ocean, alone, with two children, who had
traversed an immense cultural barrier, who had pursued and
succeeded in a career despite debilitating illness, could laugh
at the absurdity of a resident physician's sneer. And I thought
to myself, how right my father is, and how little we know of
the personal courage of individuals, particularly the IMGs.

An ill IMG, I grant you, may seem to have little to do with
the issues of personal choice and of health-care priorities that
are at the core of this book. Except for this: IMGs are the
present-day whipping boys of American medicine's frustration
with change. There is now a movement to reduce the number
of IMGs in the United States, if not prohibit them entirely
from coming here. The arguments are: there are too many of
them; their education is not up to American standards; they
take from this country and they give nothing back; we can
adjust our current physician oversupply by keeping IMGs out.
Perhaps so. The numbers, after all, are compelling. In 1993,
according to *The New York Times* (of January 24, 1996), 17,500
American medical school graduates were in training programs
in the United States and 22,706 IMGs.

But it is also important to acknowledge the dignity IMGs
possess as individuals, and to note that most inner-city medical
care, in dangerous areas and unpleasant surroundings, is done
by them, since they are willing to accept jobs that American-
trained physicians eschew. Dr. Hasan took nothing from this
country but gave instead. Ill and well, she paid her way. She
worked hard, in a field that American physicians shun, in hospitals where they do not go. Her training was different, but
her intelligence and her dedication were not. Beset by burdens
scarcely imaginable to American-trained physicians, she ap-

plied herself with vigor to relearn medicine the American way. She succeeded, unequivocally.

Policies devised for classes of people hurt individuals. Perhaps in times of crisis there may be justification for this injury, for excluding some individuals from society's largesse. But we must debate the implications and know who will be hurt before we exclude. After all, our debate might end with a conclusion that human dignity has a greater value than the lower-health-care-budget holy grail.

This country has no absolute duty to train physicians from other countries. But we do train them, as Germany trained our own American physicians a century ago. IMGs do contribute. We should know who they are before we shut the door.

One day, as I finished making rounds with the residents on the medical ward, an aide wheeled a young man through the door. Jean-Paul Pelletier was a new admission to this floor. We had expected him; the emergency room had called ahead. The diagnosis was erythema nodosum, a type of very painful allergic reaction. The young man was in great pain but did not look desperately ill. Normally I saw new patients after the residents had completed their evaluation of them. Since I made rounds every day, I would in the course of events see him the next day, but he was already here, and his problem was in my area of expertise. The residents asked me to look at him then.

There was a small problem: he spoke only French. No matter. I had majored in French at college. I could handle the interview. I began with questions that were not the foremost ones for the residents.

"Are you an American?"

"No," he replied. "French. I'm a student."

"Do you have traveler's health insurance?"

"No. No insurance at all."

"Do you have any money?"

"A couple of hundred dollars and my ticket home."

"Do you have a place to stay?"

"Yes."

"Someone with you who can help?"

"Yes."

I looked at his legs. "Typical erythema nodosum," I explained to the residents. We briefly reviewed the essentials of that diagnosis. Together we looked at his chest X-ray, ready for us in the back pocket of the wheelchair. Normal. (Some lung infections that need treatment cause erythema nodosum; we had to be certain such infections were not present.) "If we keep him here, the hospital will charge him two hundred fifty dollars a day, maybe more, which he cannot pay," I said. "He'll be in debt for years. I can write him a prescription now. If his friend will care for him, it will take a few days, a week at most, before he will walk easily again. Let's send him home now, give him my telephone number, and we'll see him back in the clinic in a week." We did. He recovered enough to head back home, where his further care was paid for by French taxpayers.

Medicaid and Medicare do not pay for foreign nationals, so the hospital bills them instead. The funny thing is, had this story been about an American student in France, the French hospital would *not* have charged.

Hélène Duval's legs were swollen, and her breath was so short she could not lie down. The veins on the sides of her neck bulged. You could see the veins pulse—a big wave, then a little one—showing that her tricuspid heart valve was stretched too wide to close. Before I had even warmed my stethoscope, I knew what I would hear: heart sounds soft and weak, with an extra sound in the middle, lub-DUB-dub, lub-DUB-dub, the meter of the word "Kentucky," the sound of a heart that has no strength left at all; crackling sounds at the bottoms of her lungs: and blowing sounds, one harsh, like an exhalation that vibrates the back of the throat, another soft, like a sigh or like blowing with the lips pursed, sounds from scarred heart valves that can no longer close. I had not heard those sounds for years. Rheumatic heart disease, a Third World disease, almost vanished in the United States, preventable, treatable. Tragic. A young Haitian woman, just recently brought to America by a vacationing couple, sponsored and hired by them to serve as their live-in maid, and so ill. I listened. I heard the sounds, as other doctors had told me I would.

Then I and the other doctors looked at her chest X-ray. Her heart was swollen to twice its normal size. The lungs were engorged with fluid. There were flecks of calcium in the damaged heart valves. This was a textbook picture of long-standing rheumatic heart disease. Which she could not have.

Because there are laws that were passed decades ago to keep tuberculosis from America's doors, potential new immigrants to the United States must all have chest X-rays before they leave home. Those with abnormal X-rays cannot come. So Hélène Duval must have had a normal X-ray. Her heart must have been completely normal less than three months earlier. But rheumatic heart disease does not progress so fast. We could check her story. She was a new immigrant to this country. It made a difference for us to know. Rheumatic heart disease can be surgically repaired. An unlikely alternative diagnosis was an extremely severe inflammation of the heart, for which we had no effective treatment. We needed to know before we made our next move.

We obtained her immigration films. The heart had indeed

been normal. Suspicious that it might be somebody else's film, we looked for clues. Same size chest. Same breast shadows. Same body fat. No telltale healed rib fractures or other scars. Same person, we concluded, except for the change in the heart. We took both films and went to our X-ray department. The radiologist on duty concurred. Probably the same person, he said, and kept the films.

Later that day he called us back and asked us to meet him in the radiology conference room. There several radiologists were milling about and a staff conference was about to begin. Ms. Duval's films were on the view board.

Taking out a clear plastic device that measures angles, the chief radiologist, grinning, pointed to the ends of the collarbones. With uncharacteristic showmanship he measured the angle first on one film—almost exactly ninety degrees, a right angle—then on the other, about seventy-five. He had not been certain at first. He had called the patient back for new films to verify that the placement of the patient, the angle of the X-ray beam, all the technical factors, were identical. His conclusion: same body size, same age person, same bone structure in almost every respect, but two different women. The immigration film was not Ms. Duval's. The angle of the end of the collarbone was the clue.

We talked to Ms. Duval about the X-ray as we readied her for surgery. She told us that she had paid a large amount of money to some men in Haiti who specialized in finding and X-raying, with a label identifying the purchaser, persons who are physically close enough in match to them to be twins, with normal hearts and lungs, so that they can use these false X-rays for potential immigrants who are ill and who then can get access to American medical care. It works, because Americans do not send treatable, dying people home.

THE CHICKEN FLIGHT

When I was a resident at Bellevue, I awaited the arrival of the "midnight chicken flight" in the wee hours of Sunday mornings. In the 1960s, Pan American Airways took tourists to Puerto Rico in the late afternoon, and the midnight flights back were cheap. These flights mostly brought immigrating Caribbeans to New York.

Bellevue residents knew about these flights. They carried ailing grandmothers, the grandmothers' nearest of kin, and a few chickens and oranges for sustenance—the chicken flight. Families came to New York to get medical care. Puerto Ricans are U.S. citizens, but they are not eligible for New York City welfare benefits until they receive Medicaid. It was hard for us doctors to tell who actually was from Puerto Rico. If the grandmother was from the Dominican Republic or Ecuador or another Spanish-speaking land whose citizens were eligible for no American services, she entered the country anyway if she was accompanied by a Puerto Rican who vouched for her.

The plane landed in New York about 3 a.m. On arrival there were immigration delays, then there was the drive from Idlewild (now Kennedy) Airport into Manhattan. We counted on the passengers' arrival about 4:30 a.m. on most weekends. We knew they would come, and we watched for them at the front door. Our first glance usually told us that the arriving grandmother was very ill. Legal immigrant or not, there was no question of sending her back. And so we admitted her to Bellevue. We understood the welfare card game. If María Pérez from Fajardo or Bayamón was last seen three months ago at Bellevue and if then she appeared to be about fifty years old, weighed one hundred twenty pounds, and had asthma; and if now the same María Pérez was seventy, two hundred ten pounds, and had heart failure, so be it. Our job was to treat the ill, not to defend the immigration system. The city hospital did not ask of a sick person her citizenship, visa, or insurance status. If and when she recovered and we found she could not pay, someone from our legal services department would investigate. It would not make a difference whether there was an investigation or not because there was never any money that the hospital could recover. The city hospital had served—at a cost to its operating budget and, eventually, to the taxpayers of the city of New York.

Pan American Airways has long since gone, but there still is the equivalent of the midnight chicken flight. When an uninsured or undocumented person becomes ill, he will still receive care, legal or not, fraudulent or not, usually at Bellevue, and the government will be the payer of last recourse.

Sometimes taxpayers say no to this underground support system. Californians voted for Proposition 187 in 1994, requiring that hospitals refuse to treat aliens. The argument had some merit. After all, the California taxpayers are paying the bills. But the argument incorrectly assumes that aliens do not pay taxes, that their employers do not pay taxes, and—most important—that no one but the person unfortunate enough to fall ill has a stake in his care.

If you are a doctor or nurse and you refuse to treat a sick person—say, a sick alien—you have to assume, among other things, that the patient is not ill with a contagious disease, also that the patient is not likely later to be found as an unconscious John Doe, with no identification, and then cost even more to treat. But the real evil of Proposition 187 is that it makes anyone with an accent or nonwhite skin a dubious person. In our society people are not required to carry proof of citizenship at all times, yet anyone with a Latin or Asian or Middle Eastern or Native American or Caribbean face, alien or citizen, born in the United States or not, is at risk of being challenged to prove his right to seek medical help.

A court injunction halted enforcement of Proposition 187.

Proposition 187 had looked very good to the legislators who drafted it and also those who voted for it. But it did not look good in the hospital emergency room in the few days that it was California law. Doctors and nurses, in a spontaneous act of heroism—some would say revolt—simply said no. As we doctors did so often at Bellevue, the California doctors and nurses refused to turn their backs on the ill. In short when required to choose between alleviating human suffering and paying higher taxes—they instinctively chose to relieve misery. "No health care for illegal immigrants" is an abstraction that is easy to say. But to look a dying, treatable Hélène Duval, or María Pérez in the eye and say, "No health care for you," is inhumane, and for good doctors and nurses, it is not easy to say at all.

THE WITCH

Moira Theodore was a witch. It was her claim, not mine. She felt strongly about this. She treasured her coven.

In truth, she looked the part: tall, anorectic, pale ashen skin, heavily powdered, dark lipstick, straight black hair hiding most of her face, like the famous Charles Addams woman in the cartoons. She always wore a long black robe and cape. She crept soundlessly—flowed, rather—into the waiting and examining rooms, tight to the wall, unobtrusive, preferring shadow. Children, glimpsing her, scurried to distant corners or huddled close to their parents. She spoke little. She was not evil—she didn't even look evil (to me), in fact, was quite pretty—and she did not enjoy frightening small children. But

she had been given powers. She had not sought them. She was
the vessel to which they had, unbidden, been consigned.

She was aware that she was different, but she was not unhappy. She was accepting, more or less, and she did not pretend to be of the world of mortals. She told me often about
her coven. Its magic, she told me, assisted in her medical care.
She was a witch, no more and no less, and she would not
permit me to treat her as anything else. My knowledge of how
to treat witches is admittedly weak—I missed that course in
medical school—but Moira Theodore was patient. She in-
structed me in what I needed to know. She sought my advice
but not my care.

Ill with a treatable but serious form of kidney disease, she
shunned medications designed for human care. She asked me
for prognoses, month by month and year by year, and she
wanted to know what might happen if her illness behaved as it
did in humans. She wanted no surprises. She wanted to prepare.
But she had strong reasons to refuse medical care. In her childhood, the sight of her mentally ill brother, in a straitjacket (I
surmised), in what she considered to be Bedlam but was probably a conventional hospital for the mentally ill, had terrified
her. To her, the boy had been tortured by his physicians, their
medicines, and their shock therapies. That her father had con-
sented to this "treatment"—possibly even requested it—had
frightened her more. She still suffered nightmares from these
events of years before. Physicians always lie, she told me; they
deliberately victimize helpless patients. She knew these things
were true because she had seen what physicians (and her father) had done to her brother. She could not ever let them,
me included, be in control of her life. She would not enter a
hospital, she said. She would take no medicine that she had
not thoroughly studied and found acceptable for witches.

Ms. Theodore was in her mid-twenties, and her mother, who

often accompanied her to my office, supported her beliefs.
Mrs. Theodore may also have been a witch. Moira told me she
was, but her mother would not discuss this topic with me.
She, too, always wore black.

Ms. Theodore once did consent to hospitalization, very
briefly, for a needle kidney biopsy. She set the conditions of
this hospitalization—how long she would stay, who would see
her, what medicines could be given, all the details negotiated
and agreed to before she came in. She couldn't afford a private
room, but we arranged for one. (She needed a dark room and
privacy for her rituals.) I and the kidney specialist agreed to
these conditions, somewhat to our colleagues' amazement and
the medical residents' disgust. I won a second consent: she
accepted a psychiatric examination that I had asked for, to
reassure me that she was mentally competent to decline care.
The psychiatrist said she was, and offered no opinion on her
ability to cast spells.

Over the course of several years I watched Ms. Theodore
die, slowly, untreated. I helped her when I could—doctored
her, I guess you could say—offering some drugs that she would
accept, trying various physical and natural-medicine tricks
when possible. We tried to make her treatment, or nontreat-
ment, a partnership—I offering what I could of my orthodox
medicine, she asking my assistance with her witch's medicine.

One summer, when her illness was worsening, she was ap-
prehensive, and sought advice from both me and her coven.
The leader of her coven had suggested that she dance naked
under an oak tree in the full moonlight. That act would cure
her, the leader said. She asked for my view. Ms. Theodore and
I reviewed the coven leader's prescription. I am generally ami-
able. Although I practice orthodox medicine, I try to help if I
can. There are limits to what I can do.

I usually spend my off-call weekends at a small country

house where my family and I escape from the city. The property is heavily wooded, with many oaks. It was a time of a waxing moon. Though I am not licensed in or knowledgeable about witch medicine, and I did not want to participate in something I am not trained to do, I did end my conversation with Ms. Theodore by promising her a branch torn from one of the oaks. I'm unskilled in botany, but I can distinguish among white, red, and pin oaks, so I asked the obvious question. The species wasn't important, she replied, she was sure any oak would do. And so, obliging, I brought her a limb of white oak—if I recall correctly—cut from the woods at my country home, in full summer leaf. The branch was more than a yard long and nearly as wide as long. The trunk of my car is small, and even with careful folding, a leaf or two dribbled out when I shut the lid.

I did not choose to witness the full moon, the nakedness, or her dance. I would not even know the correct doses: how long was the dance, for instance, or how bright the moon? I suggested that she do with the branch whatever she thought best. Witches do not smile, I suppose, but she did say, "Thank you," and seemed pleased. I don't think the oak branch helped, though. Her illness did not abate.

I used to keep on my desk an enlarged photocopy of a medical paper.* I had it framed and put it on the desk facing the patient. The paper described the case of a young Filipino woman who had been cured of very severe lupus. She had been hospitalized in Washington State in crisis—kidneys failing, multiple signs of grave disease—and she had not responded to conventional treatment. At the peak of the crisis, against medical advice, she abruptly signed herself out of the hospital.

*It was R. A. Kirkpatrick's "Witchcraft and Lupus Enythematosus," *Journal of the American Medical Association*, 1981, 245: 1937.

Several weeks later she reappeared, completely cured, fully well, having taken no medications at all. Her doctors were stunned. The woman explained that she had gone home to the Philippines, where a witch doctor had removed the curse an ex-boyfriend had placed on her. Thus was she cured.

Patients often asked me about the paper. I meant them to. I kept the paper on my desk to invite discussion about two things. First, the story tells us that there is more that doctors do not know about illness than they do know. Perhaps the witch doctor knew something that orthodox Western medicine had yet to learn. Second, the paper asks my patients to talk to me about the alternative medicines they use.

Moira Theodore knew why I had the paper on my desk; and she was candid about her alternative systems of care. The coven was only one. As Ms. Theodore worsened and her kidneys began to fail, she heard that very high doses of vitamin C would be a cure. She purchased bottles of tablets and took them. I objected: when the kidneys fail, the body fills with acid and fluid. Vitamin C is an acid, and I worried that the large amount of vitamin C she was ingesting would hasten her decline. Ms. Theodore countered my argument with her own. She had called Dr. Linus Pauling, she informed me, the winner of two Nobel Prizes and then the nation's most public advocate of megadose vitamin C therapy; he had told her that vitamin C was safe. When I protested, she had Dr. Pauling contact me directly. He told me that she should take sodium ascorbate, a non-acid version of the vitamin. I'm not very used to debating dual Nobelists, but I pointed out that the sodium in sodium ascorbate would cause her body to retain more water and harm her in a different way. My arguments were not persuasive to either him or her. She took huge doses of sodium ascorbate. But still she did not improve.

As death neared, Ms. Theodore's anxiety became more

overt. "What will happen?" she asked. "What will my death be like?" Uremic poisoning, kidney failure, I told her, would occur. I could still prevent it, but she still said no. I told her that if she continued to refuse treatment, she would gradually become lethargic. Her appetite would disappear. She might develop nausea, then vomiting. Soon thereafter she would breathe deep, sighing breaths and fall quietly, with little pain, into coma. Death would occur several days later. My news about coma frightened her. Would I promise her that, when she became unconscious, I would not take her to the hospital, tie her up, and forcibly treat her? I do not believe in assisted suicide, but neither do I believe that a physician has a right to impose his will on a patient. I answered yes, I would make that promise. And I did make it. Several weeks later she died, gently, in her mother's home, and her soul, untormented, went, I suppose, to wherever the souls of witches go.

Ms. Theodore was more flamboyant than most of my patients in her reliance on alternative systems of medical care, but she was not unique. In fact, more than 80 percent of patients with chronic illness use some form of alternative medicine. Most of them do not tell their orthodox doctors about these treatments. Certainly 80 percent of my patients don't tell me.

Yet alternative medicine, complementary medicine, ethnocentric medicine, call it what you will, is not so clandestine as it once was. It is by no means mainstream, of course, but it is not (necessarily) ascientific or even generally dangerous. Mostly it doesn't work, and it costs money. When a disease is progressive but curable, reliance on alternative medicine wastes time. Chronic disease, however, is by definition incurable, and patients get quite desperate for something that might work. Arrogance about the magnificence of contempo-

rary science is unseemly in the chronic-disease physician, and
wholesale rejection of alternative medicines inappropriate. A
number of unorthodox imports to Western medicine have
proven their worth when tested. Acupuncture, for instance,
and a variety of herbs and touch-healing methods at least palliate, if they do not cure.

Dialogue between alternative and orthodox medicine is difficult, but not impossible to imagine. Moira Theodore listened
to me. I did not convince her that I was correct, but perhaps
I was not cogent enough; she was not cogent enough to convince me that her way was best. Still, we had our conversation.

Ms. Theodore died, but somewhere there are other dia-
logues. Somewhere there are other Filipino girls talking to
other witch doctors, achieving cures unanticipated by Western
medicine. Someday we will speak a common language, and we
orthodox doctors will be able to hear what our rival, unorthodox, alternative-medicine practitioners have to say, and they,
in turn, will listen to us. We will both be wiser for the
exchange.

Meanwhile, patients' use of alternative practices is pervasive,
so much so that two senators asked the National Institutes of
Health (NIH) to create an Office of Alternative Medicine. It
is not well funded, but it has start-up funds and good ideas;
its first director, Dr. Joe Jacobs, devoted enormous energy to
his work and was very creative.

Dr. Jacobs was able to show why dialogue between alternative and orthodox medicine is difficult. Advocates of alternative medicine want immediate acceptance, or immediate
tests, of their treatments, but only under their own rules. They
distrust the scientific method and say they want common-
sense, yes-or-no answers—the treatment works or it does not.
Not controlled trials. Not gray zones. Not qualifications. Not
probabilities. Not complexity. Supporters of orthodox medi-

cine refuse to be locked into this inflexible box. Orthodox doctors have had experience with claims of efficacy subsequently proven false when placebo effects were considered, when progressive disease gave the lie to a fantasy of well-being. They trust the objectivity of blinded studies and standardized, predefined measurements of outcome. They rely on statistical probabilities. They like to know not only if but why something works.

Dr. Jacobs tried to create a common language between these two parties. He offered compromises. Let the alternative-medicine people set the rules for the use of their products; let the orthodox-medicine people set the rules for analyzing the tests. That way, if the alternative treatment really works, it will pass tests of scientific rigor and disbelievers will accept the result. After all, a large part of orthodox medicine is empirical, and, equally, not everything physicians do has a sound scientific basis. The articulate Dr. Jacobs persuaded scientists—he persuaded me—to join his effort. The public good, he said, demands that serious scientists take up this matter.

His insistence that tests of alternative medicine be done stringently enough to convince the orthodox doubters cost Dr. Jacobs his job. His arguments were not compelling enough to persuade Congress that good science and alternative medicine can live together—uncomfortably, to be sure, but trying to understand each other. The alternative-medicine advocates wanted a capitulation, not a compromise, and Dr. Jacobs' process was too slow. Since in the Washington power hierarchy a senator easily trumps an office director, Dr. Jacobs left the Office of Alternative Medicine and NIH.

Orthodox medicine has again turned its back on the effort, because the doctors are certain that if the most basic principles of good science are rejected, then they can have no conversation. But for a brief while, with Dr. Jacobs at the helm, there was a real possibility that a conversation between alternative and orthodox medicine could take place, with each party respecting the other, each committed to a common goal.

VALUES

How strongly do we value what we do? When an individual's most closely held personal values conflict with those of the larger society, which values should rule? When cost is an overriding concern, when upholding someone's personal values requires public funds, are there medical benefits we can easily do without? If you believe something strongly, will you pay to support someone else's similar—or contrary—belief?

Here are examples of situations where we must all ask—and answer—these questions:

Self-Inflicted Medical Problems

One Saturday night a police ambulance delivered to us residents at Bellevue a severely injured young man who had fallen from a great height. His bizarre garb—all black, even a black ski mask, a number of chains linked to the belt at his waist—got in our way when we tried to treat him, and it also explained his profession. He was a cat burglar who had fallen from a roof.

We could have chosen to do nothing for him. After all, his prognosis was very poor. He was not an honorable member of society. How much should society pay to repair his bones? However, no one really asked the question. Even cat burglars have families who love them. We treated him as we would any other trauma victim, vigorously, but he did die.

I will not pretend that cynical thoughts do not sometimes

occur to doctors when they treat gang members shot in street warfare, drug addicts, alcoholics, and even those who have several times attempted suicide. Sometimes our cynicism is very overt.

I once considered the case of a young man, a heroin addict, HIV-positive, indigent, and uninsured, who was admitted to our hospital one night. I heard his story the next day as I took morning report—the daily review, by a senior physician, of all newly admitted patients. The medical resident explained that by injecting himself with dirty needles, the man had infected his heart valve with a nasty fungus. There was only one cure: to cut out the infected heart valve and replace it with a new one. This would be a very unpleasant task for the surgeons, since they risked infection from HIV during the surgery, and it would be expensive, too. The residents had already called the surgeons, who had snickered a bit and made a few politically incorrect jokes. But none seriously questioned doing the operation. The cost would be absorbed by the hospital and the doctors. (This is a kind of medical socialism—the cost would show up later in higher bills charged for surgery on those who could pay.) After all, despite his eventual death sentence because of his HIV infection, the young man was immediately sick and needed to be treated now.

The real problem came several months later, when he had fully recovered. The man felt so well that he started injecting heroin once again and soon reappeared at our emergency-room door: he had reinfected his new heart valve. A different fungus, this time, but the same operation to cure him a second time. The surgeons were very angry. "How many times do we put our lives on the line for this [man]?" (they used another noun), they fairly screamed. And then, without further question, they replaced his valve a second time.

Placing a moral test on the use of our medical resources

seldom yields a clear outcome, but even imagining that a moral test is a valid way to decide whom to treat and whom not to treat tints the issues in Hitlerian colors. Think of where it leads. We could save vast amounts of money by excluding from care the drinker who crashes his car and is seriously injured; he did it to himself, you can argue, and why should we pay for his repair? Or think of the now-paraplegic motorcyclist who hadn't worn a helmet. The smoker with emphysema or lung cancer. The hunter wounded by another hunter. The mountain climber. The bungee jumper. The professional boxer. How about the football halfback with torn-up knees?

And then we come to harder questions, where cause and effect are not obvious, and it is less clear that self-inflicted harm is the issue. The sober driver who crashes while driving very, very fast. The person with high cholesterol who refuses to moderate his diet. People who do not exercise. Those who do—and injure themselves. And perhaps the most difficult of all questions: who should pay when couples bearing abnormal babies refuse abortions or when sick women insist on getting pregnant? Should children with Down's syndrome be treated when heart defects or leukemia supervene? How about the conjoined ("Siamese") twins, recently in the news, who almost every surgeon said would not survive surgery to separate them? The parents raised public contributions to pay for the surgery, sought out the only surgeon who said one child could be saved (he was wrong), and squandered the donated money, now owed for a long and fruitless hospitalization, on new cars and on drugs. An unpleasant story, to be sure, but would it have made a difference if the parents had been clean-cut honorable citizens, or if the likelihood of success had been high? Some have said that treatment of persons with sexually acquired AIDS should not have their medical care paid for with public funds. But do those who argue this way say the same of the chaste spouse who acquires AIDS from a philandering husband? Perhaps one might argue that there is no need to treat a condemned prisoner who is ill. Yet Jack Ruby, the assassin of Lee Harvey Oswald, himself the assassin of President Kennedy, was treated at public expense for his lung cancer. The fact is, there is no moral imperative so clear in these medical cases that considering it does not immediately suggest unthinkable related examples. We are compassionate human beings, and that is part of the moral equation.

Reassurance

American doctors order proportionately more magnetic resonance imaging studies (MRI) and computerized axial tomography (CAT) scans than do doctors in Canada or Western Europe. In the United States there is very little waiting time to obtain an MRI or CAT scan and equally little need to establish an order of priority among patients who need the tests urgently. But if crude death statistics tell us anything, the wide use of MRI and CAT scans in the United States does not change the overall health picture for Americans, and the figures might suggest an abstract solution: do fewer scans, and save money.

People do place value on the results of tests. Think in personal rather than in abstract terms: your teenage son suddenly develops severe, recurrent headaches. The doctor thinks that he has simple migraine, and he does not think additional tests are needed. You, however, know a young colleague who had similar symptoms, and in her case an MRI scan found a tumor, curable when caught early but lethal if ignored. You are worried that your son may have the same thing. The doctor is doubtful, but he tells you that, without an MRI test, he cannot be certain. You want the test for your son.

Or perhaps the doctor treated your colleague and wants to reassure himself. I'm acquainted with this in my own practice. For example, a pinched nerve in the neck is a very common complaint. I once diagnosed a pinched nerve in a woman who several months later began to have trouble walking. It turned out she had a very rare benign tumor in her neck and it, not a mere bone spur, had pinched the nerve. I was sufficiently frightened by having missed this tumor (it was successfully removed) that I asked the next four patients I saw with the same complaint to undergo further studies, which were both expensive and painful, before I understood that I would not likely ever again see such a tumor and that a reexamination in a few months would be sufficient to identify one if I did. Subsequent patients with pinched nerves were thus spared the second round of tests.

So who first asks for the test is not the point. The issue is: how much are you willing to pay to know that the cause of the headache is *not* a rare tumor? And who (the HMO, the insurance company, you, your doctor) should pay for it? When is it reasonable to insist on this reassurance? If you can pay out of pocket, it does not matter to you: you can obtain the test from private sources, and that's that. But should only the wealthy be reassured? Should the less well-to-do or the poor be denied equal peace of mind?

Some say doctors do unneeded tests in order to make money. Others say doctors waste resources keeping terminally ill people alive. Of course there are instances of outright fraud in medicine, as in every line of work, but in most of the anecdotes there is usually another side of the story that is less colorful but important. The expensive test you call wasteful may have excluded an uncommon but dangerous (and litigable) condition—consider the MRI for your teenage son. The patient who dies after prolonged and expensive high-technology intervention may have had a reasonable chance of recovery had the treatment gone another way; perhaps his doctors thought the costly intervention unlikely to succeed, but the patient or the family pleaded that "everything possible be done." Doctors cannot overrule a patient's expressed wish or ignore the desires of his next of kin.

Some years ago a man named George Delury helped his wife, who had multiple sclerosis, to commit suicide. Because Mr. Delury kept a diary about the suicide decision, the pain of these two people made national news. I read about it in *The New York Times* on December 15, 1995. What was remarkable about the diary is the vacillation in Mr. *and* Mrs. Delury's understanding of the state of her health, their inability to distinguish depression from realistic pessimism, and their uncertainty as to whether or not she should die by her own hand. Doctors know that such indecision is usual, that different family members often take different positions in such matters, and that they will have different opinions on different days.

From the doctors' point of view, if the patient is awake, the blood pressure is stable, and food and fluid intake and output are reasonably normal, prognosticating death in two days, two months, or two years is not possible. With uncertainty—which obtains almost all the time—they cannot refuse *a request* that a reasonable, potentially helpful action be taken. To refuse to treat when an alert patient requests help is unconscionable, and when a patient who is not alert makes (or whose family makes) clear requests for treatment, refusing those requests leaves the doctor feeling bitter and guilty, and the family, too.

Some people have suggested that doctors reserve the fancy technology for those patients who have something further to contribute to society. What exactly does this mean? High technology allows many heart- and kidney-failure patients who are important only to their families to survive. This is surely a social benefit. High-technology medicine enables us to remove gallbladders, to repair coronary arteries, to sew torn ligaments, and to correct abnormalities in unborn babies through minute endoscopes rather than through large incisions. High technology provides most of the miracles of modern medicine. A first coronary is no longer a death sentence. Very premature babies now survive. Clearly, high-technology medicine is often applied to patients who do not contribute further in any way or who nonetheless die. But when the technology is used, the outcome is seldom known.

The End of Life

"Would somebody kill my cousin? Please?"

That's what Dudley Clendinen seemed to ask, but did not, in an Op-Ed article that appeared in *The New York Times* on February 5, 1996. Mr. Clendinen disliked the way we treat elderly people. It is not that we ignore the elderly, he said, but that we are too attentive. He was unhappy that doctors kept his cousin Florence alive too long. At the age of ninety she had tried to kill herself but failed, and she lived on for three more years. The nursing home cost her life savings. Once or twice in those three years she got pneumonia, and the nurses, Mr. Clendinen complained, gave her antibiotics, sent her to the hospital, and she survived.* His cousin "wanted to die," he wrote. "The System wouldn't let her."

---

*His attribution is probably wrong. The nurses may have been authorized to use their discretion, but most state laws require that antibiotics be ordered by physicians.

Mr. Clendinen's argument is common: that doctors, nurses, and the whole medical-care system fight against all logic to save those who cannot be saved. "The System," nameless and faceless, orders that elderly sick people be kept alive no matter the cost and no matter the pain. It is abstract, under no individual person's control, just a noxious, ineffable presence to rail against.

Though his anger was obvious, Mr. Clendinen proposed no solution. He wanted *somebody* to do *something*. But *some-* is a nebulous prefix. The *-body* should be named and the *-thing* to be done defined.

Several facts in his article make me disbelieve that his cousin Florence "wanted to die" and that "the System wouldn't let her." For one: after her suicide attempt, she remained clear of mind, and we are not told that she tried again or asked her family or her doctor to help her die. She had signed a living will that did not prohibit administering antibiotics to her. To a doctor, this antibiotic issue is important. Swallowing a pill is a trivial, nonpainful act. For a doctor not to prescribe antibiotics is not a passive decision but a specific choice, not all that different from denying food or water. Doctors do sometimes make that choice. I have—for patients in irreversible coma, or moribund ones. But Florence was alert, conscious, and able to speak for herself. She could have refused the antibiotics. She did not.

What if, in pain or discomfort, Florence asked for help? Most laypersons who believe that doctors force treatment on unwilling patients are themselves confronting this situation for the first time. They may not know that patients who say once that they want to die often change their minds. "The System wouldn't let her"—this implies that the System said, "Do not act. Let nature take its course." But I do not see it that way. "To abandon" is an active-voice verb. "To kill" is, too. The question Mr. Clendinen might have asked is this: Who will kill Florence? Who will look in her alert eye and say, "I will not treat you. I have decided that it is your time to die"?

Florence had two sisters, Bessie and Carolyn, both of whom suffer from dementia, but neither is dying. Bessie and Carolyn are, in the *writer's* word, "terrible." We do not know that they agree, since they are demented, but Bessie and Carolyn may not feel their lives are "terrible." They may still want to live. And it is not Mr. Clendinen's place to infer that his cousins want to die.

The System is made up of individual doctors and individual nurses who have faces and names. They make decisions for both the short and the long term. An abstract System cannot act. An abstraction cannot abandon and cannot kill. *Somebody* makes a choice. There is always personal responsibility. Who of those in the System should kill? Mr. Clendinen might have taken this responsibility himself. He might have returned Florence's pill bottles. Many patients take overdoses, as she once had. If death were truly her wish, he could have helped her try suicide again. He did not. Other patients on their own stop taking their medicines and let their diseases run their course. She did not, nor did he suggest that she should.

He might have taken her home. He might have had her transferred to a terminal-care hospice. He could have selected another set of caregivers. Dr. Jack Kevorkian is not everywhere, but there are physicians who are willing to withdraw more than machine support when there is no hope—withdraw food, for instance, or medication. Mr. Clendinen might have considered mercy killing. Courts almost never prosecute for murder when four criteria are satisfied: the person was, in fact, dying; there was no hope of recovery; the person clearly asked to die; the killer had no motives of his own, such as personal convenience or money, that influenced his choice. From the way that Mr. Clendinen presented Florence's case, the first three criteria were not met; we do not know about the fourth. He asked the wrong question. The real question is: Can we Americans afford to care for the very old? If the answer is no, then we should engage executioners. We should not ask doctors and nurses to do that work.

What a monstrous option! Executioners! My presentation is surely harsh. However, the idea of willfully killing the elderly (phrased passively: "let them die") is not new. The argument has been voiced by sincere, compassionate people. Legislators and budgeters also raise the issue in veiled ways. However, to utter the words is different from accepting the idea. I have chosen my side: as a doctor, I do not choose the function of executioner; as a person, I believe I have a moral contract to protect those who gave me life. Euphemisms, abstractions, and the passive voice soften the heinous idea but change none of the facts. To withhold basic needs from conscious, sane people requires an action. For one person to ask another to "let her die" is not abstract. An action requires an active-voice verb. A verb requires a subject. In this case, the subject is "who," and the verb is "kill."

A few days after Mr. Clendinen's Op-Ed article, *The New York Times* published five letters to the editor, two from physicians and three from laypersons. Both physicians pointed out that Florence was alert and capable of making her own decisions, that predicting precisely when death will occur is nearly impossible, and that Mr. Clendinen had substituted his impression whether her life was worth living for that of his cousin. And the lay writers all accused the medical profession of insensitivity to death with dignity. One of them even stated that she (the writer) had a friend who wanted to die, but who "let herself be seduced by a medical friend"—note the passive voice—to accept further treatment! Is it not arrogant to presume that the dying woman had not decided to live?

Doctors and laypeople are talking past each other. Physicians focus on day-to-day decisions, and they see patients vacillating. They know that prognoses are uncertain. Families remember who the loved one once *was* without seeing that he or she still *is*. But there is opportunity here for meaningful dialogue.

Evan J. Kemp, Jr., spoke to this concern from a different vantage point. Disabled himself, he charged in an Op-Ed article in *The Washington Post* on January 5, 1997, that DNR (do not resuscitate) orders, enacted to *protect* patients against intrusive medical care, are instead being used to coerce disabled patients to surrender their rights to receive care. He cited an instance in which a patient who had agreed that she would not receive *extraordinary* resuscitation in the event of sudden death or coma, was tied to her bed to prevent her from stealing food from other patients' plates because, when she signed the DNR statement, the hospital staff stopped giving her food and water! At the time this was published, a Supreme Court case on doctor-assisted suicide was pending. Mr. Kemp clearly saw that, whether from economic or work-reduction motives, permitting physicians to kill can quickly move from killing at the patient's request to killing for the family's or doctor's *or HMO's* convenience, when the family doctor, or HMO, not the patient, judges the patient's life to be unsatisfactory.

Other Priorities

Medical care costs too much and takes up too much of the federal budget, we say. We must find savings somewhere.

I do not accept the first part of that assertion. Whether medical care costs too much or too little is a matter of the priorities a society sets. We can make health care a high national priority and increase its budget, or a low priority and decrease its budget. We might give a lower priority to defense spending—after all, the world is now putatively safe from global war—or a higher priority when war threatens once again. We could save on agricultural entitlements. Or space exploration. Social Security. Education. Welfare. Transportation. Parks and museums. Congressional staff. Environment. There are myriad alternative priorities and alternative budgets we as a nation could choose. There is no preordained ceiling or floor for health-care expenditures. There is only that which we are willing to pay. There is only the value we assign to our personal health.

Keeping people alive and well costs money. Letting people die is cheap. Looked at by the crude measure of the cost of medical care, a child who dies of asthma costs less to society than does one who recovers and repeatedly returns to the hospital over many years. A soldier who spends years in rehabilitation costs more than does one who dies on the battlefield. A woman whose kidneys fail, then partially recover, so that she no longer needs dialysis, needs more medical care than if she had died in the initial illness. The premature baby who suffers brain damage but survives continues to add to the nation's medical bills for decades. Smoking-caused illnesses are expensive, but if smokers die early they do not collect Social Security, so it is cheaper to let them die. (If cost were the only issue to consider, the writer Richard Kluger has pointed out in his work on tobacco, the Surgeon General might ask more people to smoke!) If we truly wanted to save money, we would exert no effort to save patients with poor prognoses. In fact, we are doing this now, when HMOs refuse to consider giving their patients access to experimental treatments and when states allocate care according to cost-effectiveness criteria. It would save vast amounts if we refused to treat those who no longer contribute to the national good.

The Third Reich notwithstanding, it is beyond my imagination to believe that this nation will ever choose to save money by letting people die untreated. I pray that we never even consider that a debate on such a premise is valid.

Each thing we value has a cost. How much is your choice— to have the MRI scan for reassurance, to replace the heart valve of an HIV-infected heroin addict—worth? But, you may argue, no one has asked me to assign value to reassurance. No one has asked me to price care for the elderly or the disabled. The complaint is legitimate. You have not been asked, directly, to perform this calculus. But you have been asked, indirectly and generically, to say yea or nay to the following: Medicare costs are too high and must be reduced; do not waste money on worthless technology; get rid of "inefficiency" in the medical system. If you have responded yes to these, you have assigned values.

In medical care, an alternative term for "inefficiency" is excess capacity, but to eliminate excess capacity is to eliminate easy access, rapid delivery of services, and, above all, personal choice. If you do not have the choice to get that MRI scan for your son's headaches, because only persons meeting specific criteria are eligible to be scanned, and your son does not meet those criteria, the system is more efficient. If your mother with chest pain can no longer receive treatment near her home but has to be transported to the cardiac-care center seventy miles away, then the system has saved the cost of supporting an intensive-care unit that is only partly used. England spends one-tenth of what the United States does for intensive-care-unit beds, as *The Washington Post* reported on March 9, 1996, but critically ill patients in Britain are taken from one hospital to the next in search of an available cardiac-monitoring ward, CAT scanner, or surgical intensive-care unit, which some English now consider a crisis. New Yorkers did not tolerate transport of critically ill patients to MRI scanners just a few blocks across town. Improving efficiency seems like a very good idea—your personal inconvenience, after all, costs your insurer little—unless you place value on convenience and on your ability to choose. Which do you prefer? Redundancy and choice at higher cost, or economy with no choice? Are you comfortable if a stranger makes a judgment on the value of your or your relative's life, then uses that judgment when deciding to shorten or to sustain that life? Or would you like to make that choice yourself?

These are choices. We do have value systems. The value systems do have worth. The cost of our values should be placed on the table. We should be asked: How much are our values worth? How much are we willing to spend?

When we examine our values, we may find that our current health care is a bargain.

3

WHO IS IN CHARGE?

DISAGREEMENTS BETWEEN PATIENT AND DOCTOR

My office was being renovated, and carpenters, plastic sheeting, and dust were all over the place. I stood in front of my secretary's desk, the two of us trying, not successfully, to contain chaos, when the telephone rang. My secretary hunted beneath the plastic, found the instrument, and answered. She listened a minute, then handed the receiver to me, telling me that the caller, a gynecologist colleague of mine, known to us both for his unflappability, sounded worried.

There is not a lot of chitchat when doctors interrupt one another in midday, and my colleague is by nature taciturn. He made his point immediately. "I have Ella Redgrave in my office with me," he said, the *r* rising from deep in his throat, vowels broadened by his Belfast birth. "I think she has a pleural friction rub. She's supposed to fly to Paris tonight. Can you take a quick look at her?" I thought: Not many gynecologists carefully examine their patients' lungs, and then I thought: Quick looks are never quick. Oh, well. My office was closed because of the renovation, so I was free, and I could examine her in a colleague's room nearby. I asked him to send her over.

Ms. Redgrave's name was well known. I had seen her, off and on, for several years, treating her for a very mild form of spinal arthritis, an illness rare in women. Now thirty-three, she had had a couple of episodes of short-lived disability from which she had recovered completely.

Ms. Redgrave worked on projects throughout the world. She had been born in London, but it would be hard to say that she had an actual home. Boston, New York, Paris, and Stockholm were places where she could be reached most times. When she called for an appointment, it was usually from one of those cities; when she was in New York, she usually stopped by, to say hello or to talk about a new symptom or to renew a prescription. One time she asked me to sign medical papers and take an X-ray so that she could become an American citizen. This particular time I had known she was in town for only one or two days. She had not made an appointment to see me, just one with her gynecologist, perfectly routine.

She had heard a sound in her chest. She had asked some Harley Street doctors in London about it a few months before. One had diagnosed nasal polyps, another asthma; they had given her treatments but the sound remained. She was suspicious, so she mentioned the sound to my gynecologist colleague. He dutifully listened to her lungs. He thought it was a friction rub, a noise like two pieces of leather rubbed together, indicating inflammation or injury to the lung's lining inside. I disagreed. I thought the sound was a localized, low-pitched wheeze. On both sides of the chest, scattered about, high and low, wheezes of different pitches suggest asthma, but a wheeze on one side, in a single place, low in tone, raises a different concern: air cannot get past an obstruction. Why is the airway blocked?

Ms. Redgrave, normally rushed and hyperkinetic in speech and style, was in a mild frenzy that day. She was booked on an evening flight to Paris and had an afternoon of preparations to complete. Even Paris was only a stopover for a day or two, and then she would head for Africa—Nairobi, maybe, or it was Brazzaville, or Lagos, I don't remember anymore—where her new project was about to begin. She expected to stay wherever it was for many months. In New York it was now about noon.

I sent her for an emergency chest X-ray. Half an hour later she brought it to my office. I flipped the film onto the viewing box.

I do not think I gasped audibly, but I was stunned by what I saw—enough so that I double-checked the name and record number on the film, the body size, the amount of fat, the breast size, the bone structure, and all the other features that doctors use to confirm that an X-ray belongs to a specific patient. There, in the middle of the left lung, about an inch across, was an irregular, dense shadow: cancer! Instinctively I scanned the bones for metastases, and the lymph node areas for signs that this tumor had spread. I saw none. I felt a wave of nausea pass. Everything was wrong about this. Thirty-three. Nonsmoker. Female. Unbelievable.

Ms. Redgrave's manner was informal. Amidst the dust and the plastic sheets, she sat cross-legged on the floor, waiting for my comment. I held the X-ray for her to see. "I'm sorry to do this to you this abruptly," I said, pointing to the ominous shadow, "but we don't have a lot of time for discussion. It looks like lung cancer. There is no reason you should have this. It could be something else, but we have to find out as soon as possible. I don't want you to go to Nairobi. I would like to call a chest surgeon, here, now. Or in Boston, or London or

Paris, wherever you would like to be treated, but this cannot wait for your return."

She asked me to call a surgeon in New York. I reached our hospital's best at once, and he agreed to see her right away, for he was between operations. After looking at the X-ray, he immediately sent her for a more definitive, special type of X-ray, one that usually was done only by appointment, but he had it done within the hour. The new films even more clearly said cancer, still no evidence of spread. It was now about three o'clock.

Ms. Redgrave can make decisions quickly. She made a few telephone calls from my office, hunting under the plastic sheeting for the telephone. We scheduled surgery for early the next week, and she set about to rearrange her affairs.

The next day she called to see me again. She said her father, even better known than she, had flown in from overseas in his private plane. Could I discuss her situation with him, please? They came to my office together. It was a bit surreal, this world-famous face with a world-famous name sitting on a packing box, construction debris on all sides, his daughter squatting cross-legged on the floor at his side. Her personal support systems, people who could visit and be there to care for her as she recovered, were better in Boston, they decided; my chest surgeon friend made a call to a colleague of his there.

A few days later, in Boston, the tumor was removed, and I did my daily rounds with Ms. Redgrave by telephone. She turned out to have a rare type of cancer, one not associated with smoking, and unrelated to her arthritis. I heard the operative findings from the surgeon first. When the pathology report came back the surgeon called again, then she did, then a rheumatology colleague whom I had asked to look in on her, all within the space of about an hour. All seventeen lymph nodes were negative for cancer. It had not spread—and could be cured. Ms. Redgrave recovered quickly. Then, delayed by three months, she began anew her peripatetic career.

The renovation of my office was complete and my office was once again clean. One day, the receptionist called to tell me that a delivery was heading my way. In a few minutes a tall man in full livery—a well-tailored gray uniform, peaked cap, high leather boots, discreet family crest on the left breast pocket—walked in. Not your normal deliveryman, he was a personal courier, direct from London. He handed me a small package, accepted my signature, bowed, and left. The package contained a lovely book, elegantly bound in leather, with a gilded stamp of the same family crest, and on the flyleaf a handwritten, nearly illegible, note of thanks from its author, the young lady's father. This wonderful, unique gift would have been perfect, had I not, deciphering the inscription days later, realized that I had been given a book intended for the Boston doctor. I assume he received one inscribed to me. I wrote a thank-you note, of course, but I did not point out the error.

"It's a touchy situation," my obstetrician friend told me. "Sandra Richards is another doctor's patient, and he thinks she is fine, but I think that she has something in your field and needs treatment. She's fourteen weeks pregnant. Her blood count is only half what it should be. I'd like you to see her, but I don't want to step on her doctor's toes.

"Here is what I have done," she continued. "I'm going to admit her to the hospital to do some tests, though I know the tests could be done in my office. If she comes into the hospital for a day or two, I can ask you to come by to see her as a teaching consultation, because of your lupus pregnancy study. Then you can tell me if I'm off base or not. Just be a little sensitive to her primary physician, please, and don't delay her discharge too much, or the Utilization Committee will be after me."

I had worked with this obstetrician before. She has very good judgment, I knew. If she thought there was a problem, there was likely to be a problem. On the other hand, in the fifteen or so years I had worked at the hospital, I do not think that I had ever spoken to Mrs. Richards' primary doctor, a very senior physician on our staff. He had a fine reputation and a mostly office practice that included many donors to the hospital. He rarely had patients in the hospital, which is why I ran into him so little. I knew that he himself had been ill. I thought he had perhaps even retired.

It did not make much difference to me that Sandra Richards was someone else's patient. As a salaried staff physician in the department of medicine, I had a lot of teaching duties. I and my salaried colleagues often saw other doctors' patients (with their permission, of course) for the purpose of teaching physicians in training. Sometimes private doctors asked us full-timers to do a teaching consultation because they thought the students would be interested in seeing a particularly unusual case; sometimes they asked so they could impress their patients with their personal roles in the medical school; still other times they asked for teaching consultations to get unofficial opinions for which the patients would not be billed. (Usually they did this last one to save the patient money, but sometimes just because they were cheap.) On occasion, as now, the point of the teaching consultation was to get a new opinion without seeming to—a subterfuge that worked especially well when two doctors disagreed about what to do.

I was at Sandra Richards' bedside within a couple of hours, and she was expecting me. She was a bouncy sort who laughed a lot, chatted a lot, perhaps a little nervously, and moved a lot around the room. A young lawyer—I do not think she had yet taken her bar exams—she was well informed, and she knew that she was very anemic—had been for a couple of years, she said. Her doctor had told her that she had "chronic mononucleosis," and she had accepted that (unlikely) diagnosis without dispute. She lacked energy because of the anemia; otherwise she felt well, she thought. Sometimes women with pregnancy complications are very frightened, but she was cheerful and optimistic. Her pregnancy seemed to be normal, and she was excited about it. It was too early for her to have felt the baby kick, but she was expecting that any day.

Mrs. Richards did not know that the severity of her anemia threatened her baby. A mother's severe anemia means that the baby may not get enough oxygen during its period of most rapid growth, and may be hurt, possibly suffering brain damage, as a result. I knew, but she did not, that to protect the baby something had to be done—and soon.

Pregnant women often develop heightened color in their cheeks. That blush, or glow, is what Mrs. Richards and her doctor thought explained the rash that had recently appeared on her face. They were wrong. She was too anemic to have the pregnancy glow, and to my trained eye the rash said lupus. Subway diagnosis, I call it, the type of diagnosis you can make across a crowded subway car. Mrs. Richards' case history was so typical that it almost parodied a textbook description of lupus. Yes, she had had arthritis. Her doctor had attributed it to mononucleosis. Chest pains, ditto. Swollen glands, ditto. Low white blood count, ditto. Low platelet count, ditto. Admittedly, her symptoms were mild, on the subtle side, but her doctor had to have been asleep to miss this diagnosis. His error did not make much difference when Mrs. Richards was not pregnant, because her illness was so mild that it needed no treatment, but she had not been checked for complications, like kidney disease, and she had not been watched very closely, as she should have been.

I ordered the necessary laboratory tests, then I called Mrs. Richards' obstetrician from the nurses' desk. The obstetrician had anticipated what I would say. She would call Mrs. Richards' primary physician, she said, but would I please talk to the patient and her husband if I could? She would make rounds between seven and eight that night and would herself talk to them then. Would I be around? Perhaps we could meet them together?

When several doctors have unpleasant news for a patient they care for together, they usually decide beforehand who will be the first to broach it. I had left Mrs. Richards' bedside a few minutes earlier telling her I wanted to clear up a few issues with her obstetrician before I gave her a report. Now I went back to Mrs. Richards' room. I told her that I had talked to her obstetrician, who had asked me to discuss my conclusions with her. She thought her husband would arrive shortly, and wanted to wait for him. I had other patients nearby whom I needed to see, so I went to see them, and when I returned, Mr. Richards was there. He was a lawyer, too, which I knew, but if I hadn't, his pinstripe suit and his yellow, lined legal notepads, poised at the ready, would have made it clear. Young lawyers are eager. They like to record all the facts.

"I don't think it is mono," I began. Then I launched into a litany of the facts we had, what else we needed to do to be certain of my tentative diagnosis, what the alternative diagnoses might be, and what lupus was like. I gave them some pamphlets about the disease and about being pregnant when one has it. "Be wary of television and the tabloids," I said. "Lupus shows up in doctor shows a lot. When a famous person has it, newspapers and television tend to dramatize it. A few years ago a New Jersey youngster with lupus was kidnapped.

To force her release, newspapers and television vastly over-stated the seriousness of her case. They terrified lupus patients for hundreds of miles around. Don't assume that what you hear is correct. Call me to check it out.

"Your case is fairly mild," I went on. "Mom is basically okay, and, at the moment, the baby is, too. But we need to treat Mom to protect the baby." Then I began litany number two, which was about cortisone and its side effects.

Mr. and Mrs. Richards were not as surprised as I thought they might have been, having had a suspicion that something was wrong, something more than mono. Mr. Richards was as upbeat as his wife. Both saw mostly the positive side of things. Whether that was their nature or whether they were unable to accept that Mrs. Richards was ill was not clear to me. (The former, it turned out.) They asked a lot of questions. I ex-pected them to—they were lawyers, after all.

With cortisone, Mrs. Richards' blood count would improve in several weeks, I told them, but that was too slow to protect the baby. We therefore gave Mrs. Richards transfusions to raise her blood count to normal quickly. Her energy improved dramatically, and then the cortisone took effect. Like many patients first being treated, Mrs. Richards said she had not realized how ill she was until she felt better. The pregnancy continued normally, and Ruth Richards was born at full term.

Mrs. Richards' doctor asked me to take over her care, and then, as it happened, he retired. When I talked to his replace-ment—I knew him fairly well, a recent graduate of our residency program, newly on our staff—he assured me that he would look to see if any other lapses in care might have occurred. The Richardses had considered suing because of the misdiag-nosis. But in the end they thought the care she had been given was sad, not venal, and it had not caused lasting harm. Both Sandra and Ruth were well. The Richardses did not sue.

Ella Redgrave's and Sandra Richards' first doctors were wrong in their diagnoses. Misgivings led to further evaluations, new diagnoses, and new treatments, which changed their lives. In both cases, the health insurance policies were flexible enough to allow them to seek second opinions, and both patients took advantage of that flexibility.

How would these people have fared with systems that use gatekeepers or closed panels of physicians, that offer no freedom to seek further care? The success of these systems depends on meeting three criteria: first, the primary physician always makes the correct recommendation, from which all subsequent recommendations flow; second, the necessary expertise to deal with the patient's needs is available within the closed system; third, the initial diagnosis is sufficient for deciding (without recourse to appeal) on the next steps. Both Ms. Redgrave and Mrs. Richards would have been badly served by such an arrangement. Without access to alternative diagnoses, Ella Redgrave would have been treated for asthma, and the baby might have been permanently harmed.

Closed panels, and gatekeepers, work well for commonplace problems and for illnesses that heal themselves, and most fevers and rashes, coughs and diarrheas, get better on their own. Lacerations that need suturing, sprains, and ordinary fractures also can be handled by most doctors. Closed panels and gatekeepers are also wonderful when prevention is the goal: vaccinations, blood pressure and urine checks, mammograms and screening for various other cancers—all these are unquestionably done better by managed care organizations than by fee-for-service medicine. Also, sprains, lacerations, and common fevers present little opportunity for a patient to think that the doctor is wrong.

But in more complex cases, when things are not going well, the patient may have an opinion that differs from that of the primary doctor. The problem is that gatekeepers and closed panels do not permit *the patient* to decide that another opinion is necessary. Since referrals and second opinions cost money, the accountant's opinion prevails. With gatekeepers and closed medical panels, the criteria for protecting the patient are not met. There must be more flexibility. Sometimes the patient, not the doctor, is right.

I should point out that HMOs do not use the word "gatekeeper" but instead speak of the "family" or "primary care" physician, who knows the patient (and the family) well, and who decides when to refer to another doctor. This system can work—if this primary-care doctor really is the patient's doctor. But consider the following story:

In one HMO, a patient had a complex problem. Her primary-care doctor, Dr. A, arranges for her emergency hospital admission one evening. At the point of admission, a different family physician, Dr. B—then rotating according to an on-call schedule of the HMO's devising—assumes responsibility. Because inpatient doctors working in hospitals also rotate on day and night call, a third physician, Dr. C, takes over in the morning. This inpatient rotation changes each week; the patient was admitted on a Thursday night; and on the weekend, starting Friday night, new daytime (Dr. D) and nighttime (Dr. E) doctors are in charge of her "primary" care.

At each change of shift, the physician who is leaving (for instance, Dr. B) gives an oral account of pending problems to the physician coming on call (for instance, Dr. C). If Dr. B does not mention a pending problem to Dr. C, Dr. C may pay it no heed. Indeed, if not called by the nurse, Dr. C may not even visit the patient on his shift, and may not pass on information to Dr. D.

In one case I know of, the patient had five separate "primary care" physicians—sequentially, not simultaneously—during her first three days of hospitalization. A consulting physician who knew her well was not one of the five, and he could not assume care unless by invitation. A catastrophe ensued. When I saw the records (as part of a legal quality-of-care review) my first question was: Who is this woman's doctor? because I truly could not tell. The five doctors were interviewed: none considered himself to be her primary physician while she was in the hospital.

In 1988 a New York State Hospital Review and Planning Council (the Bell Commission) recommended that a limit be put on the number of consecutive hours that resident physicians work in hospitals, lest they be too tired to make good decisions. Senior physicians, in some organizations, have adopted the same limited-work rules. The intent of the Bell Commission recommendation is laudable, but the result is what happened here: no one physician takes charge. If the patient wants a long-term plan, when follow-through is critical, when doctors-in-charge change every twelve hours, to whom can the patient plead?

A MORAL DILEMMA

I do not like guns. I have fired one only a few times in my life. Once was when a friend's father set out as targets scraps of paper on a big rock in his backyard and let his son and my brother and me fire a .22 rifle at them. We were about ten years old at the time. Thrilled as I was, I was appalled at the danger, and I understood how young I was. Not knowing much about the relative softness of lead or stone, about energy absorption and dissipation, and trained by comic-book pictures of dashed lines tracing ricochet paths, I imagined deflected bullets killing us all. We survived the day, however. Lead squishes on rock. A .22 slug hits a rock and falls straight down in a crunched little heap.

Several years later some friends of my parents invited me to shoot skeet at a farm in Vermont. This was fun, but I missed the little disk every time and prayed with each shot that no innocent bird would fly by. The kickback of the heavy shotgun hurt my shoulder. I had little desire to shoot skeet again.

A third time was when I had a job one summer in which I had to dip gray steel shotgun and rifle barrels into boiling sodium hypochlorite to make them turn gunmetal blue: an interesting, but hot and rancid process for a kid in high school taking chemistry classes. When the barrels were "blued" I had to test-fire each one, which I did into a safety box. I used a standard carpenter's hammer instead of a firing pin, placed a cartridge in the back of the barrel, placed the barrel in the box with cartridge end sticking out through a little hole, and whacked it hard. Boom. Then I opened the box to see the results. We didn't use ear protectors in those days. The noise and smell were very unpleasant. Also, when the barrels ruptured in the safety box, which they sometimes did, it was a mess and I'd have to clean it up.

But the main reason that I don't like guns is that I believe that a living body, human or animal, is a magnificent machine, and what guns do to it is senseless and loathsome. I don't even like being around guns. So it was natural that I did not look forward to Peter Malone's visits to my office.

Pete Malone was an undercover police officer, a special agent of some kind, not a city cop. He might have been FBI, I didn't quite figure out the details. He had a type of arthritis that occurs mostly in young men and causes the spine to stiffen and hurt. In severe cases it forces its victims to bend forward, to walk looking at the ground. The disease is called ankylosing spondylitis, or poker spine (as in "stiff as a poker"). To look to one side, Mr. Malone had to swivel his whole body around at the hips, because his spine, from pelvis to skull, was for all practical purposes like one solid bone. I thought it would be hard for Mr. Malone to squeeze his back tight against a wall, pistol drawn, glance sideways with only the slightest motion of his eyes and head, sight a miscreant, jump out and yell, "Freeze!" as undercover agents always do on television. Overall, however, he was not very disabled. Stiff as his back was, he could do things that most men could do.

Ankylosing spondylitis also causes a type of eye inflammation called iritis, in which the iris, the colored part of the eye, becomes inflamed. Vision can be nil during an attack. Bouts of iritis, untreated, can last days to months, but treatment can stop it within a week or two.

Mr. Malone had not gone to a police surgeon for treatment because he did not want a record of his illness to be in his file. It would have cost him less to go to the police surgeon, but it was worth it to him to pay out of pocket to keep his secret from the department, or bureau, or whatever it was he worked for. "I love my job, Doc. I don't want them to take me off the street," he told me. At his request, on each visit I gave him my promise that his records would remain confidential.

The reason I did not like his visits was the ritual he went through each time he came. Since I usually examined all his joints, he usually stripped to his shorts. He was not modest; he did not ask me to leave the room while he undressed. My small examining room contained only my writing table, two chairs, and an examining cot. Mr. Malone carried a lot of police hardware. When he undressed, all the hardware came off and he put it on the table, right under my eyes. Handcuffs, badge, and some sort of combat knife first. Then came the chest gun, leather harness and holster, followed by the bullet belt from his waist. Finally he reached down, with some difficulty because of his back, and unstrapped a stubby little gun from his ankle. All that horrible stuff on my small table gave me no room to write. I was very careful not to knock his equipment off.

Most of the times I saw him, Mr. Malone was well. He would come to get his medications refilled, for me to do some blood tests, to measure how his back moved, to see how well he could fill his lungs with air, and to chat about how things were. The visits were casual and bland, except for my distaste about the lethal equipment that ended up on my table, which I kept to myself.

A normal New York summer is hot and muggy—people get edgy. The summer of 1977 was worse than most. Anxiety was high that year. Even on hot nights everyone stayed indoors. A serial killer, called Son of Sam because of the enigmatic signature he placed on the otherwise baffling notes he sent, was stalking young women—mostly in Brooklyn, mostly in romantic places—and shooting them point-blank. He had been killing since the summer before. I think the count of his victims was six at the time. The city was near panic.

I was not thinking of Son of Sam when Mr. Malone arrived one day that summer. I focused on the problem at hand. It was obvious from his dark glasses, and more obvious when he took them off, that Mr. Malone had iritis—now for the first time in both eyes. He had had bouts of iritis once or twice before, and this was clearly his worst episode.

"Working awful hard, Doc," he said. "Fix me up quick. I got to go back in a couple of hours."

"What are you doing?" I asked, fatuously.

"Son of Sam," he answered. "I'm on stakeout, eighteen

hours a day, in Brooklyn. Got to get back on the job. Can't let my boss know I'm like this."

"Can you see?"

"I can see enough. I won't shoot anybody. When I'm like this I won't fire my gun."

I started to hallucinate about random Brooklynites being killed by a heavily armed, stubborn, blind cop who mistook them—many, many of them in my hallucination—for Son of Sam.

I had been in medical practice for seven years, but I had not yet faced any particularly discomfiting moral dilemma. This seemed to be one. I had made a promise of confidentiality to Mr. Malone many times. But now I asked him to reconsider the secrecy, to take time off, to do something to get him off that job. But he said the police force was using every man it had, every man was on overtime, they were calling in extra police from all over the Northeast to find Son of Sam before he killed again. Eyesight or not, he was needed. And he loved his job.

I did not know any way to get his sight back quickly to normal, so I called an ophthalmologist with whom I worked from time to time and who had seen Mr. Malone before. She thought she could get his sight functional within a few days, so I sent him over to her. And I worried.

I talked to my hospital's administrators, who talked to the hospital lawyers, about what was the best thing to do. They hemmed and hawed but eventually said that patient confidentiality took precedence over a potential risk to public safety. After all, they reasoned—then I reasoned, too—he was only one of hundreds of police officers hunting Son of Sam. It was unlikely that he'd be the only one to be presented with a clue that could lead to capture. In any event, we expected that he would be able to see well again in a few days. And Mr. Malone had promised me that he would not fire his gun(s) if he could not see. I was not happy—in fact, I was miserable—but I accepted their advice.

A few days later, Son of Sam was caught, not in Brooklyn, but in Yonkers, at the opposite end of the city. Pete Malone was not part of the arresting team. No shots were fired in the capture. Eight million New Yorkers slept better that night. One of them, me, slept best of all.

A doctor's moral dilemmas may be an interesting topic, but it is not the topic I want to focus on here. The point is: Who owns a patient's private information? There are many discussions in the press, on television, in Congress, about privacy—of HIV tests, for instance, or about testing for genetic flaws. The public debate on this topic is vast and far more profound than anything that I can marshal in these pages. But I want to focus on one overlooked aspect of the issue: do recent changes in health care change the privacy rules?

In the 1970s Mr. Malone had the option to purchase his own, private medical insurance and to bypass the insurance provided by the police. He exercised that option. You don't have to agree with his motives or with my assent to his request to understand what he did. You can be very upset that he chose to work in his dangerous profession while he was disabled, but there were other ways to deal with that choice.

If Mr. Malone's supervisor had noticed anything amiss, he could have—should have—required a fitness-for-duty examination. Airline pilots, long-distance truck drivers, even doctors have to undergo these on reasonable request. In a fitness-for-duty examination there is no doctor-patient relationship; the doctor, selected by the employer, is unambiguously the employer's agent. If the employee chooses to lie, so be it, but the doctor is prepared, and the patient knows the rules of the game. The operative words here are "on reasonable request." The employee patients are not required by law voluntarily to incriminate themselves. (They might be morally so obligated.) Doctors in a private relationship with a patient—such as I had with Mr. Malone—must not be informants to someone else. But doctors in a fitness-for-duty examination are in a different position.

What if the employer has a health plan for his employees that gives no choice of providers and then, exercising his economic power over the provider, demands private information about an individual employee? What if the employer requires, as part of the contract with the provider, that the latter regularly report confidential information? What if the doctor, wanting to please the party that pays, volunteers "tips" to the employer about whom to hire or fire?

The scenario is not far-fetched, and it is not unique to today. When I was in military service in the mid-1960s, I did health-status examinations of coal miners in West Virginia in order to compile statistical data; it had nothing to do with personal care. We invited miners to come in for examinations: almost no one did. It was not my northeastern manner and speech, or the British manner and speech of my supervisor, both strange in rural West Virginia, that kept the miners away. Rather, a few years earlier, one of the large local coal companies had required its miners to have chest X-rays "to be sure you are okay" and had then fired, without compensation, those found to have black lung disease. The miners assumed that my team had been hired by the coal company and that our arrival in town represented round two.

In company towns, absolute power belongs to the companies. Are company health plans so different? If a doctor's services are purchased by the company, does that put pressure on the doctor to be the advocate of the company and not the patient? Does the patient understand the rules of the game? Does he know for whom the doctor speaks?

Clearly, people like their employers to pay for their health care. I certainly do. But we have to be careful about what rights we, as patients, surrender, and about what we expect our doctors to do for us or against us. As a doctor, I would not mind displaying on my office wall a disclosure form—sort of like the Surgeon General's warning labels on cigarettes—that says how I am paid and to whom I must give the results of your tests. It is fair that patients ask me those questions. It is obligatory that I answer them.

Mr. Malone understood the validity of his contract with me, and I honored that contract. I also understood my liability, or at least my guilt, if he had not kept his promise, if he had fired his gun, if he had killed innocent Brooklyn residents as I feared. What we both understood was a principle: if I could have told his supervisor about his eyes, I could have told another supervisor that his employee had a cancer of which she was still unaware, telling the supervisor to save himself the health-care bill, to fire the employee before she found out. Or AIDS. Or a genetic disease. Or anything expensive.

It's a tough problem. Do you pay your own doctor's bills? Are you sure that you know for whom your doctor works?

4

CENTRAL PARK

Seen from afar, from high up in a skyscraper, Central Park sits soft and organic within a hard, geometric gray world. Seen from nearby, Central Park is more diverse: trees with concrete, city with forest, join in proximate harmony. Within the park's borders there seems to be no city, only grove. The park speaks to the passerby.

The park's ancient rock, of origin in Ordovician time, thrusts through the soil. Like a caul, earth slips away. There are grooves in the rock, carved by glaciers tens of thousands of years ago, when there was no city, no human dwellings. Immense dark mass beneath the stroller's feet, with surface scratches that antedate civilized man, the rock whispers: The city is transient on the bulk below, rock is timeless, you are not, nature is stronger than man.

Walkers in the park do not mostly think in geological time,

I suppose. They have narrower thoughts. "Am I late?" Or "What was that noise?" Some people cross the park in fear. To many, the very name Central Park means more than rocks and trees. It brings to mind two young women, one a jogger, the other a musician, both savagely beaten in this place. The two women now have public names: "the Central Park Jogger" and "the Central Park Victim." Their stories are horrifying: their bodies were invaded, first by attackers, then by doctors. We hear of them and we think: It could be my wife's body, or my child's, or mine, lying in a strange place, poked, prodded, and violated by strangers. And no one knows her (or my) name.

The first news accounts of these horrors focused on the violence and anonymity of the crimes. The next spoke of medical miracles about to ensue. One account of the Victim's injury, by Malcolm Gladwell and published in *The New Yorker* in July 1996, praised modern trauma surgery. If all trauma victims had the high quality of care this woman received, Mr. Gladwell remarked, recovery would be commonplace. But even so the story had an ambiguous end: the Victim's father was seeking a good rehabilitation center for his daughter. The story did not say whether the Victim recovered or whether a medical miracle had really occurred.

Melissa Poggi did not acknowledge my introduction, for she was in coma.

Her morning had been ordinary. Nothing strange until she fell from her chair. The details of what happened then were confused. One witness said she fell forward, another said backward. One said she struck her head, another that she did not. She either had had a convulsion or had not. If she had, the convulsion had begun either before or after she fell. In the end the details were not important. What was important was that her co-workers saw her lying on the floor and called 911. An ambulance took her to a nearby hospital.

Melissa Poggi had suffered a stroke. But a stroke at the age of thirty-two? Friends said, and tests confirmed, that she had not used cocaine or any other illicit drug. The emergency-room doctors searched widely but found no obvious cause. Blood pressure, arteries, heart, the usual places where one would find something that might explain a stroke at a young age were all normal. Too rapid clotting of the blood, then? The answer to that question was yes. An abnormal antibody had caused her blood to clot and the stroke to occur. The doctors began treatment to prevent new strokes, but the treatment did not work. A few days later Ms. Poggi suffered a second stroke.

One small part of the brain determines whether a person wakes or sleeps. In Ms. Poggi's case, the first stroke had damaged that part. And another part of the brain, where speech arises, was the site of the second stroke. Four days earlier she had had an ordinary morning. Now she was sleeping most of the time. When awake, she did not speak.

Her doctors asked for my thoughts, so I went to see her that night. I was not encouraged by what I saw. Yet she is young, I thought, and young people have the power to heal. The amount of damaged brain tissue was actually quite small: brain swelling may have made the damage seem greater, and I guessed she would improve when the swelling went down. Since I was testing an experimental treatment that I hoped would prevent more strokes, I offered to transfer her to my hospital and my care. Her doctors and family agreed. Because unstable comatose patients need neurology special-care units, I asked a neurologist colleague to work with me. The chairman of our neurology department was unhappy about this when he heard of our plan.

"Don't you understand," he challenged my colleague and

me, "that she'll never talk again? That she'll never wake? That we will never get her out of here? Her insurance will run out," he continued, the voice of a chairman whose department will surely be blamed by the Utilization Committee. "She is already receiving adequate care. Let the other hospital eat the bill."

I might have listened to him. He had, after all, written a textbook on coma. He had given the name used for Ms. Poggi's condition: persistent vegetative state. Patients in this state are unconscious though their eyes are open. They are unaware of people or things—or so doctors think, but who really knows? They do not answer when spoken to. They sleep most of the time.

I disagreed with the chairman. I expected that the brain swelling would subside, and if she had any chance of recovery, I thought, it would be in our hands. I ignored his advice. Ms. Poggi came to our neurology floor.

Months later, I would like to say that I now know Melissa Poggi, but that would be untrue. I know superficial things about Ms. Poggi. I know the biology of her disease. I know that she is pretty, with straight blond hair and pale blue eyes. That she smiles sometimes. That she cries. That when her eyes open and we hold up signs she does not respond. I know that sometimes she follows people with her eyes. Does she see a person, or only changing light and shade? Is it a reflex or is it human thought? That I do not know. She does not talk. She sleeps. From her parents and from her fiancé I now know something of who she was. I have learned about things she once did and once hoped to do. I watch her sleep. Mostly I look for medical signs to which I might make some intelligent response. Sometimes I hope, by powers I do not possess, to draw forth her thoughts and dreams, if think and dream she does. Now and then, when her eyes open and she looks my way, I introduce myself again, tell her where she is and why, tell her small details about the day. There is no sign that she understands this monologue.

The experimental treatment worked—to a point. She suffered no more strokes, but her damaged brain did not repair. A doctor's first rule is: Do no harm, but our treatment violated that rule. We had placed a large needle into the big artery in her groin in order to wash her blood. When we removed the needle the artery leaked. Her thigh filled with blood, swelled to twice its normal size, and turned black and blue. That caused pain. Worse, the leaking blood became an abscess. We drained the abscess and caused more pain. We placed plastic tubes into her veins. She pulled out the tubes, so we tied her hands. The first abscess caused a second, leading to more tests, more surgery, and more drains. I heard her scream. Did the scream mean that a vestige of personhood still remained? Animals scream when they are in pain.

Patients in a persistent vegetative state raise complex issues. One is, when does one withdraw treatment? Another is, what constitutes "consent" to do so? Doctors do not agree on these points. Some doctors say that the responses to pain do not indicate human awareness but are only automatic reflexes, pointing out that even mollusks, insects, and worms avoid pain. Some doctors believe that patients like Ms. Poggi are technically dead and that it would be justifiable to let them go completely, and to remove their organs for transplanting to others.

Ms. Poggi no longer has intravenous tubes. She does have a feeding tube that goes into her stomach and another tube in her bladder to drain her urine. She wears a diaper. She is now haggard and skeletal. Her once long hair is short, to make grooming simple, but even so her grooming does not last for long.

The neurology chairman was right. Melissa Poggi will not likely converse again. She may not waken. Princes do not come to the beauties who sleep on neurology wards. Her family has not told me that they know what her future will be like, but I believe they understand. As the news story said, the parents are seeking a good rehabilitation hospital for their daughter.

Normal life is not often possible after severe brain injury. Yet we doctors do treat these patients. And we do raise hopes.

Science creates miracles, yet scientists fear for the future of science, saying that Americans are scientifically illiterate and equate pseudoscience with true science, that America will suffer because people who do not understand science cannot interpret or master the world.* Only if Americans accept the primacy of science, the argument goes on, only if nonscientists become excited about science, will the nation advance. Failing that, we will not be competitive but will sink into superstition and magic. Scientists offer remedies, change the national mood. Television shows, movies, and books should portray them as heroes, and we should teach science's excitement and relevance in the schools, advertise its success. The very thrill of science will seduce the public, they believe, will improve the commonweal, increase research funding, and lead to a better America.

*See B. Alberts, quoted in *The New York Times*, December 7, 1995; Carl Sagan, *The Demon-Haunted World: Science as a Candle in the Dark* (New York, 1995); M. Angell, "Shattuck Lecture—Evaluating the Health Risks of Breast Implants: The Interplay of Medical Science, the Law, and Public Opinion," *New England Journal of Medicine*, 1996, 334:1513–18. But see also the counterargument that science is well respected and well funded in D. S. Greenberg, *Washington Post*, July 8, 1996.

I am sympathetic to that argument. But the public accounts, like those of the Central Park Jogger and Victim, already suggest more success than has been the case, suggest that science always works. Mostly it does. But medical science has not yet solved all problems. Not all hospitals offer good services, and not all brain-injured patients revive. That "the parents are seeking a good rehabilitation center" also means that recovery has not occurred. Scientists and reporters stay silent on this point. Scientists cannot tell us what the Jogger, the Victim, or Melissa Poggi will be like one or two or five years from now.

Scientists brag that science is self-correcting and they do not publicly discuss error. A scientist whose theory fails says, "Of course," and in good fellowship withdraws. Failure is an occurrence to transcend, and there is no need to apologize, no need to dwell on failure's meaning. It suffices to say, "We used to think such and such, but now we know so-and-so is true." Failure is openly discussed only when spectacular events so require: an explosion of a shuttle flight, a warped space mirror, a physician who forges clinical trial data, AIDS not yet cured.

We cannot thoughtlessly boast of medical science's success when its weakness is so apparent to Ms. Poggi's family. Fifteen months after she first fell ill, Ms. Poggi recovered partial speech. She could say some words and follow some directions, but conversation was minimal. She had almost no control of her movements. She was confined to a wheelchair, unable to feed or bathe herself, though able to control her bowel and bladder. In this day, damaged brains do not fully heal. Today's molecular biology, designer drugs, and gene transplants will not make her normal again. For the sleeping beauty who today occupies our hospital bed, science offers no magic kiss.

While proclaiming science's successes, scientists must also understand that promises which they cannot fulfill in the near future harm their cause. Science *can* boast about what it has already done—its attainments are vast—and at the same time acknowledge that there is much yet to achieve. Science's arguments are compelling only when its protagonists openly declare that science has many strengths but is not divine, that science's successes are great but so are its failures, that (for the moment, at least) there is no power to help Ms. Poggi waken or speak, that nature may always be stronger than man.

PRIORITIES OF DOCTORS, PRIORITIES OF PATIENTS

One day I met Alison Reza, twenty-three years old, tall, pretty, mature, cheerful, confident, athletic—overall an attractive young woman. Alison had had bothersome but not frightening symptoms for about five years. Rashes came and went, especially when she went to the beach. She lost a little hair one year. Her glands had swelled. Sometimes her joints hurt. She tired more easily than her friends did. Another doctor told her she probably had lupus, and I agreed.

I spent two hours talking to her and her parents, announcing to them Alison's future lifetime of illness, doctors, and medicines—not an easy concept to accept at that age. We talked about her symptoms, her diagnosis, what her options were, what her life would be. I had had this type of conversation many times before.

First discussions with patients are important. I try to be as open as I can with the information I have at hand. I am comfortable telling patients if the doctors disagree. For those who want to delve into the matter more deeply, I offer the scientific papers that support my opinion and, to be fair, sometimes those that contradict it. And I like patients to tell me what is on their minds.

The talk with Alison should therefore have been easy for me. It had required no genius on my part to confirm the diagnosis. Alison had already sent ahead to me, before her visit, the important laboratory tests, and my message would be fairly optimistic under the circumstances. Alison's case appeared to be mild, her prognosis very good. As I saw it, there were other reasons to be hopeful. The family seemed close and concerned. Alison was mature enough to deal with the problem on her own. She had already read the Lupus Foundation's brochures and was well informed before she came. The family knew about the worst possibilities. I could reduce rather than add to their dread.

But after the Rezas left, I felt ill at ease. Why? First discussions with families are always fatiguing, but Alison's problem had been straightforward and well understood, I thought, on both sides. I empathize with people like the Rezas, but even so, discussions of this type do not normally upset me. Driving home, I asked myself: What was missing? After a while I realized two different parts of me had been talking to the Reza family, but they weren't talking to each other.

One part was a practicing doctor with nearly thirty years' experience caring for young women like Alison. The second part was a scientist, recently head of the government agency that funds most of the nation's research on lupus, overseeing every bit of government-sponsored research being done on that disease. In the consultation room, the doctor and the scientist should be speaking the same language. What frustrated me was how little of the scientist in me I had used, or even could use, in my doctor talk with Alison and her family. Of course, I could and did talk about animal models of lupus, about new theories, and about new treatments on trial. I could also talk to her about life choices and about living with illness. But I did not share with the Rezas my awareness that those latter topics, the social and emotional effects of disease, are barely researched, do not attract and often repel scientists, who consider them messy subjects unworthy of serious study. Down deep, I was uneasy knowing that scientists do not care about the details of Ms. Reza's life.

Biomedical research scientists, like most of us, depend on someone to pay them for what they do. They compete for research grants. In the national competition, ideas, unrelated to pragmatic issues, win the game. "Good science" wins the game. And what is "good science"? It includes high quality of course, imagination most certainly, and deep knowledge. Curiosity-driven science, *undirected* science, science in which only the scientist judges what is worth examination, is good science. Strategic, goal-oriented science, science in which larger societal purposes are acknowledged, is not good science. The patron of strategic, directed science is industry, our best scientists argue; the patron of curiosity-driven, good science should be government.

I find a dissonance in this argument. Government supports curiosity-driven science because taxpayers have *granted* freedom of inquiry to the scientists. But a grant is not an entitlement. It is a gift that can be withheld if the public need is not served. Scientists sponsored by government grants disagree. They become angry if the grantor tells them what to do. Direct my science, they say, and it will no longer be good, curiosity-driven science. But doctors have a different view. Faced with patients like Alison, they would prefer to see *patients* set at least part of the research agenda, to have the agenda relate more closely to Alison's problems.

So would some powerful members of government, it turns out. Representative John Porter, chair of the House Labor/ HHS Appropriations Subcommittee, asked in 1995, "if the nation will have enough resources to maintain the current model of NIH—one spreading money widely, calculating that a few successes will finance or justify the general investment." He raised the issue of "a more directive approach to research, [with] funding allocated only for particular purposes." He questioned the assumption that *only* scientists have a stake in choosing what science is good or what is eligible for federal largesse.

Doctors ask scientists to consider patients' priorities, but scientists mostly heed their own, ranking the value of research by the elegance of the science, the possibility of a clean solution, and the question's importance in biology. Primary causes and mechanisms of disease merit study. Relief of symptoms does not. Specific human suffering is of lesser priority.

It is efficient when scientists choose their research topics freely. By all measures, tax dollars are well spent in this way. Serendipity arising from good, undirected science has given us cures and prevented diseases far more often than has targeted research. There are inefficiencies in targeted research: the science may not be ripe, or the scientists' minds may be too mundane. But as a doctor, I see gaps in our medical knowledge, and in our opportunities, that the scientists do not see, and I believe they should be thought about.

Scientists and doctors do not think alike. Science students wanting to go into medical research ask me about the merits of taking an M.D. or a Ph.D. degree. The difference, I explain, is that Ph.D.s do research on topics or problems that are both interesting and soluble. To them, the absence of a good theoretical base in a problem's solution is "black box" stuff—magic, not science. M.D.s have their topics thrust at them by patients, by human life in all its diversity. Ph.D.s can walk away from human questions that are excessively complex, but M.D.s must deal with whatever comes through the door, even if there is no likely solution. For the man gasping for breath, it makes little difference whether the doctor sees the problem as intellectually exciting or not, so long as his breathing can be eased. For a doctor, the patient's clock, another person's calendar, dominates his day. I must correct this abnormality by such and such a time, or the patient will die. The scientist has his own clock—and much more control: I must beat my competitor to the answer and find the solution before my next grant application is due. M.D.s address immediate needs: someone is suffering—do something now. Ph.D.s face future ones: What is the root cause of this illness? Will knowing the cause lead to a cure? From the doctor's point of view, elegant science is nice when you can use it, but pragmatism rules.

Driving home after my conversation with Ms. Reza, I began to understand that the supposed dialogue between doctors and scientists is not a colloquy at all but a one-way, hierarchical monologue. As I saw it that night, doctors want to talk to scientists, but the opposite is not true. The scientists are not listening.

Some scientists don't even listen on the hospital wards. "Don't tell me what you think the diagnosis is," I have heard scientists tell clinicians. "I will do my new test and *I* will tell *you* what the diagnosis is." They have no need to see the patient, no need to have ever seen a patient with the disease in question, and certainly no need to have seen the patient in the earliest phase of the illness, when the symptoms were ambiguous and the patient was just beginning to ponder the possibility that her whole life was about to change. The clarity of science. The messiness of having to apply science to a real person.

You can learn a lot about the monologue if you go to medical lectures. Mostly, scientists talk and doctors listen and take notes. You see the notepads and you hear the questions at the end. Flashbulbs pop and camera shutters click: some of the doctor listeners photograph the projected slides. Others use tape recorders or videocameras. They try to understand the molecular biology, the genetics, all the technical details of the talk. Some sleep, of course. In other lectures scientists talk to other scientists, or doctors talk to doctors. But lectures by doctors that scientists listen to are rare.

It is an attitudinal thing. It has to do with intellectual hierarchy, one-upmanship. When scientists rank-order intellectual achievement, they place their own at the top and disdain clinical knowledge. As a rule, they do not expend much effort trying to understand what doctors do. They may try to understand some parts, to learn the tricks of diagnosis, for instance. After all, to apply a molecular biological test to a disease, you ought to agree that those so diagnosed fit its criteria (even if you can't define those criteria yourself). Scientists also select anecdotes from the doctors' lexicon to make their lectures livelier (they would say more *relevant!*) to students or the public. But when it is time to listen to the doctors' priorities or even to concede that the doctors' viewpoint has worth, they often demur. It is easy to be dismissive when you don't have to talk to Alison and her parents.

Sometimes, feeling churlish, I make this point to my colleagues. Once, I tried to change the situation. One—a close friend, actually, and an elegant scientist—wanted saliva specimens from patients with a disease in which saliva does not flow. Scientists who never see patients often ask for specimens from the patients of doctors like me who do. Sometimes the inconvenience to the patient is trivial and sometimes it is not. In this case, my patients would have to spend half an hour, an hour, or more trying to produce enough saliva for my friend's test. I told him I'd make the request of my patients only if he told them face to face what he wanted to know, and then sat with them as they spat. He did this, annoyed, of course, but he got my point. Specimens come from real people who are willing to inconvenience themselves for research, people who want and deserve to be told what is happening and why they are contributing their time (and saliva). Meeting my friend, listening to his explanation, and then to my less jargon-laden translation of his explanation, the patients understood more about their disease and were happy to spit for him.

Doctors and scientists have common goals. Both hope to prevent or cure disease. The scientists have absolute aims— all or nothing, prevention or cure, no halfway measures. The doctors are compromisers. They settle for a little improvement here, a little comforting there, more time, and avoidance of doctor-caused disease that is the side effect of a treatment. Of course, doctors will welcome a new cure, but until the cure or prevention is at hand, being able to give comfort or to predict future trouble will have to suffice. It may even save money. (Think of the savings if we could delay the chronic illnesses of old age, Alzheimer's disease, for instance, for just a few years.)

It is paradoxical that scientists take pride in the rigor of their methods but are selective in the topics to which they apply that rigor. Once I returned to my home from a peer-review meeting—where scientists ranked grant applications submitted by other scientists. I felt that evening very much as I had after talking to the Rezas, but angry, too. Most of the applications discussed at the meeting had been based on bench science (with test tubes and animals) rather than on clinical science (with patients). Some applications had both. I was frustrated that the bench scientists required no stringency of clinical skill.

You have to know that scientists are very snobbish about the journals where they publish their findings. Some journals are considered high-quality. If an applicant has published ar-

ticles primarily in these journals, he wins points. Other journals are low-quality. The *Journal of Clinical Investigation*,
which despite its title publishes almost no clinical science,
counts as high-quality. The *Annals of Internal Medicine*, a clinical journal read by practicing physicians, is, for the purposes
of grant application review, low-quality, because it publishes
very little bench science work. A second point to understand
is the very formal style of scientific articles: introduction,
methods, experimental results, discussion, and conclusion. To
see how rigorous the author has been, one always studies the
methods section.

Back from the peer-review meeting, I spent a day in our
medical-school library surveying all that year's high-quality science journals that contained the word "clinical" in their
names. I found that the methods sections in their articles usually filled more than a page with details of laboratory technology, but *without exception*, the section describing patients (the
clinical science part) was appallingly brief, often only a single
sentence such as "We obtained blood samples from thirty patients with X disease." There were no definitions of diagnostic
criteria, no discussions of the duration or severity of disease,
age, treatment, other health problems, or anything that true
clinicians consider to be critical to understanding patients.
The scientists who edit and who read the high-quality journals
apparently considered rigor in clinical science irrelevant—is
"clinical science" oxymoronic? Clinical physicians, knowing
the complexity of diagnosis and the instability of day-to-day
variation in a patient's health, find the casualness an outrage,
as did I on that day, fifteen or so years ago. It hasn't changed.

Doctors know that diagnostic criteria require judgment, the
sorting of small facts, and they know that how you ask a patient a question can determine its answer. Doctors understand
that personality and social context and age and ethnicity gov-

ern disease perhaps as much as or more than do cell membrane proteins, cytokines, and regulatory genes. Scientists find all this uncertainty messy. They eschew clinical engagement, even as they readily accept a clinician's statement that this person has lupus and that this one does not, without questioning how the clinician reached that conclusion. Worse, they scorn the value of clinical expertise. "It is not intellectually interesting. If I can't measure it cleanly," they seem to say, "it is not worth knowing."

As a youth, I greatly admired an essay by the French poet and essayist Paul Valéry, an imagined conversation between Socrates and his doctor, Eryximaques. Socrates, ill with headache, painful arms and legs, dry mouth, agitation, and extreme fatigue, frail, not himself, is puzzled. If he were the world's most intelligent man (Valéry said it more elegantly) yet depended on the doctor to return him to health, did not that mean that the doctor outranked him in intellect and in value to society? "If you show me that you know me better than I do myself," Valéry had Socrates say, "ought I not to conclude from this that all my effort is puerile?" "It is true," Eryximaques replies, "I know what is in your heart and between the bones of your wonderfully endowed skull. I can tell you that you will be better tomorrow. But what you will do when you feel better, all the wonderful surprises you have to offer, all that escapes me." And he continues, "If you knew what I knew, you could not know what you do know." In other words, everyone is a specialist in something. I, Eryximaques, specialize in returning bodies to health. You, Socrates, specialize in building philosophy. To Eryximaques, the two disciplines, philosophy and medicine, are not hierarchical. They are parallel.

I know that scientists, more likely than doctors, will eventually find keys to our major scourges. They will prevent and cure them. And for that reason scientists are right to vaunt their prowess. But scientists and doctors work with different calendars. The former look to the (often distant) future, the latter are firmly rooted in the present, where there is no hierarchy, just difference. Science and medicine are parallel, not ranked. Side by side, not one above the other.

When something exciting happens in science, we scientists and doctors and science administrators want to boast of it. We call press conferences, issue news releases, give interviews. Reporters always ask, "Is it a breakthrough?" and "When will there be a cure?"—natural enough questions, since the answers are important to their readers, auditors, and viewers— to patients. We scientists and doctors and science administrators generally reply, "Yes, a breakthrough." Why else would we have announced it to you? Even though we have no means of prognosticating the future, we often say, "Ten years to a cure," far away enough in the future so that no one will remember, we hope, if our estimate turns out to be wrong.

Science gives us insight into the biology of illness. The recent progress in understanding disease has been extraordinary. Consider lupus. When I was graduated from medical school, half of lupus patients were dead within three years of their diagnosis. Today 90 percent are alive and well at ten years, and almost as many are alive at fifteen and twenty years. One of my patients called me today, mostly to brag about her son, but mentioned that it was thirty years since she had been first diagnosed. (She was upset about being forty-six.) Most lupus patients now marry, have babies, and lead reasonably normal lives. Each decade, each half decade has seen startling scientific advances, "breakthroughs" about lupus and about other diseases. For lupus, the breakthroughs in the 1960s were anti-DNA antibodies and complement. Then B and T lymphocytes. Then antibody subtypes and affinities. Then HLA types, cytokines, cell-cell communication, and molecular genetics. Each advance has led to a promise that a cure would be forthcoming in less than ten years.

Once, the only drugs we had to treat lupus patients were aspirin and nonsteroidal anti-inflammatory drugs (NSAIDs)—hydroxychloroquine, prednisone, azathioprine, methotrexate, and cyclophosphamide. Today we have aspirin and NSAIDs, hydroxychloroquine, prednisone, azathioprine, methotrexate, and cyclophosphamide.

The last two sentences are not misprinted. No word-processing error or computer glitch here. We are indeed using the same drugs now that we used thirty years ago, not magical new treatments. Why, then, do lupus patients do so much better?

There are several reasons. Probably the most important is that clinicians, not basic scientists, have learned to understand the disease better, to anticipate its problems better, to stay their hands when new symptoms do not require treatment, to be aggressive when ominous signs appear, and to tailor their treatments to maximize benefits and to minimize side effects. Another reason is that advances in other fields have helped patients with lupus: better drugs to control high blood pressure, better antibiotics, better intensive-care units, and better kidney transplants. Most of these advances have come through small steps, not breakthroughs, and through clinical experience as well as from research. Clinicians are open-minded enough, even eager, to apply findings of the biology of one disease to that of another. Some of the successes with lupus do derive from advances in the new biology, and clearly visible on the horizon we can see developments, "breakthroughs," that may lead to a cure. We do not in truth know whether these will come in five years, or ten, or never. But the prognosis for lupus patients continues to improve, because *both* clinical science *and* basic science have improved. There is no hierarchy here.

Science and medicine are parallel, not ranked. Side by side, not one above the other.

I once disagreed with my superior, a basic scientist, on this topic. We were discussing what projects to fund if my institute's budget were severely cut. I said that we were funding much high-quality, highly ranked, but duplicative research. I gave examples. "I would opt for diversity," I said. "Skip some of the duplication, pay for something not in rank order, choose it because it brings a new idea to the table and because it is important to patients." "No," he countered. "The duplicative studies should receive priority because they are good science. If you bypass them, you choose poor science." Use only the criteria of other scientists, he seemed to say, while I was more willing to use my own judgment (I had the authority—I was head of our institute at the time) developed over three decades as a practicing physician. We had different priorities, the scientist and the doctor.

It was these different priorities that disturbed me the evening after the Rezas left my office. As a scientist and administrator, I had been quite proud of the progress we have made in understanding lupus, proud even of my own contributions to it. As an institute director speaking before Congress, I had boasted of our achievements in our studies of lupus. But as a doctor I saw then and see now a breach between the science and the medicine, which leaves me, in my doctor mode, able to talk effusively to Alison Reza about what I will be able to do for her ten or twenty or fifty years from now but speak only vaguely, in generalities, about what I can do now. I worry that the scientists' hubris and inflexibility prevent introspection, and that they will not be flexible enough in their choices of research topics or humble enough to consider priorities other than their own.

IS MEDICINE A SCIENCE?

My reflex expletive was too loud. I had hoped I was considerate (the small night-light, not the big lamp, lit my book), but my shout woke my wife.

In his book *The Demon-Haunted World*, Carl Sagan had written, and I had read: "Museums that claim to be about science are really about technology and medicine." And: "There's . . . a fair amount of medicine and technology [on TV], but hardly any science." His book argues for increased scientific literacy. Medicine and science are different, he says, implying a syllogism that goes: Science is good and great; medicine is not science; therefore medicine is—what? unimportant? irrelevant?

Though I apologized for my yelling and my wife went back to sleep, I did not sleep at all. The casual polarization of medicine *or* science had angered me. Science's defining criterion is its methods, Sagan wrote, but to be a scientist does not require formal training. If you observe, analyze, and predict using data, you are a scientist. !Kung San tracker-hunters, Sagan says, observe data (animal tracks), analyze data (How long ago were the tracks put down? The animals are heading in what direction? How many animals?), and make predictions (We will find the herd at such and such a place). They are scientists, he says. Chimpanzees sticking reeds into termite mounds to find a meal practice science. Doctors do not?

One credo of science is that facts do not change. Physical data define what is true. Dispassionate analysis of these data prevails. Prior truths can be counted upon. Truth is obvious when different experiments or different data sources give the same answer. Create a hypothesis. Test it. Test it again from a different point of view. If the result is always the same, the science is good, and the hypothesis will predict outcomes. Data will grow to facts, the only absolute.

Medicine's methods are those of science. Medicine also has prior truths, known physiologies, and known experience (what specific symptoms imply). It uses independent evidence. A patient describes his symptoms. The doctor forms a hypothesis (diagnosis). X-rays, blood tests, physical examinations, patients' outcomes, and patients' opinions are the independent data sets that test the hypothesis. Medicine does make predictions: the prognosis, the prediction as to what a treatment will do.

Laboratory scientists generalize their experiments when they publish their results. Similarly, on the basis of generalizable experience, doctors predict a course for an individual patient. And similarly a !Kung San tracker-hunter uses implicit general principles to track, like a chimpanzee stalking termites.

The question that made me shout aloud—Is medicine a science?—troubles very few, but it does trouble me. The implication that science's truths are absolute and medicine's are not is a false one. In truth, scientific fact, no matter what the discipline, is relative, *not* absolute. Facts do change. And there are hierarchies of truths.

Hierarchies? Scientific truths that change? The very idea makes the most garrulous scientist mute. Yet the relativity of truth is not so strange an idea to understand. Consider the following very public tales. The legal proceedings in the cases of David Baltimore and Teresa Imanishi-Kari, like those concerning O. J. Simpson and others about silicone breast implants, have been widely reported. It is not my intention to review the legal issues or the details, but to show that what "truth" means to you very much depends on your prior experiences. Is there only one version of truth? Whose version of truth prevailed?

A postdoctoral fellow in a research laboratory (call her scientist A) accused her immediate supervisor (call her B) of lying in a scientific paper. The supervisor's supervisor (call him C) sided with B. A highly public battle ensued. The details of the experiments themselves were quite arcane. An independent review panel concluded that sloppy record keeping and different interpretations of the same data explained the dispute.

Daniel Kevles, a writer sympathetic to science, described the events in an extensive interview with C, concluding that the real dispute was between pedestrian and inspired science. Genius, he wrote in *The New Yorker* in May 1996, consists of ignoring the untidiness of ordinary data to see the larger picture beyond, while small minds focus on details. The truly gifted scientist need not distinguish weeds from saplings in order to see that a forest lies ahead. For a genius, it is proper to discard inconvenient data if the larger purpose is served.

A man stood trial for the murder of his wife. Scientific blood DNA evidence pointed to the guilt of the accused, for samples of blood taken at the crime scene matched his. To prove the match, a police officer had taken a sample of the defendant's blood. But the officer failed to account meticulously for its whereabouts at all times thereafter, and the jury acquitted the defendant.

Scientists were appalled. To them, the best scientific evidence ever presented to a jury had been conclusive, and it had been ignored.

Nonscientists saw the verdict differently. Science had not

been on trial. A man had been. Scientists had seen, or had differently valued, only one issue: whether the murder-scene blood matched that of the accused. The answer was yes. But the jury, I surmise, saw two issues. Which is more probable, the jury asked, that the DNA evidence proves that the defendant was present at the scene of the crime or that police officers sometimes forge blood samples to close a pending case? Scientists had not considered the possibility of fraudulent samples, but the jurors did.

In the early 1990s, the doctors of several women ill with scleroderma, lupus, and rheumatoid arthritis believed that silicone breast implants had caused their diseases, a proposition with which their patients agreed. True, the women might have become ill even without breast implants, and no one knows the cause of these diseases. Also, if implants cause disease, women with implants ought to fall ill more often than do women without. But no one knew the facts. No one knew how many women had had implants. No one knew what their health was like a year or two or many years after the implants.

The government had several new studies done. The answers? We were told that the results of the new studies "fail to support the hypothesis that exposure to [silicone breast implants] is associated with a significant increased risk of development [of these diseases]."* What does that sentence mean? Its language is medical language. Passive voices, negatives, qualifiers—prototype doctor-speak. Translated into common

---

*M. Hochberg et al., "Lack of Association Between Augmentation Mammoplasty and Systemic Sclerosis (Scleroderma)," *Arthritis and Rheumatism*, 1996; 39:1128.

English, the sentence means that implants are (probably) safe, that implants (probably) do not cause disease.

Analyze the text more deeply. Read between the lines. Contrast the sentence with plain syntax: "Silicone breast implants do not cause scleroderma." The doctor-speak is purposeful. "Fail to support" is a negative, uncertain assertion. It does not precisely mean "refute." The "hypothesis" is a tentative, incomplete thought, not an established one. "Exposure" suggests that, under different conditions, silicone implants might be safe and that women might not be exposed to risk. "Is associated" means that if you can point out a flaw in the methods of the study, if you can devise a better experiment, if you can develop better statistics, you might show a different result: the tests done are not conclusive. "Significant" is a jargon term, to which I'll return. "Increased risk of development" is an unconfident notion, different from causation; it also opens a window: the risk may be below our ability to measure. "These diseases" narrows the conclusion: it acknowledges that unnamed diseases are still possible.

Doctors do not use plain speech. They write in medical jargon for a reason: scientific truths are relative, not absolute. Science cannot prove a negative. Science cannot prove that an implant does *not* cause a disease. "Truth" in science is defined by a statistical test. "Truth" exists when there is less than a 1-in-20 chance that an experiment is wrong. Scientists express this chance as a percentage. The probability (p), they say, is less than 5 percent that we are wrong (or more than 95 percent that we are right). Sometimes scientists are more rigorous: they set p at less than 1 or less than one-tenth of 1 percent. To a jury, if something is 95 or 99.9 percent likely to be true, is it true enough to convict?

I think juries worry little about the statistical question. They worry about the relative one: in this day, in this time, what is wise? Did—do—juries, frivolously or maliciously, ignore science's truths? I doubt it. I suspect instead that they decide that scientists are not asking the right questions or enough questions. This is an irony, since failure to consider all possibilities is a signal of scientific ineptitude. Juries on breast-implant cases had been asked: Is it *possible* that, in *this* particular woman, silicone caused her disease? Did the implant manufacturers try to protect her? Was she fairly warned? Scientists answered : It is unlikely that implants cause disease. I believe lawyers call that answer nonresponsive.

Mavis Green huddled in the corner of her bed. Small, looking younger than her late teens, she mumbled her replies to our questions. We could not understand her. We heard rural Jamaican patois—*h*'s weaving in and out of words in the wrong places, the woof and warp of her speech randomly placing aspirates where we did not expect them. Her anxious eyes darted from one of us to the next.

Ms. Green's temperature was very high. Spherules of sweat rolled slowly down her brow. A thin transparent green tube forced oxygen into her nose; its elastic band pushed her hair into her eyes. Her pulse was rapid, and her breath came in short gasps. Wires under her gown tethered her to a bedside monitor, which in turn cheeped each frenzied beat of her weakened heart. We saw her swollen joints. We took out stethoscopes and listened to the sounds of that heart. Low, rumbling, "cchhhwwuuuuúp-d'-d'." That meant the mitral valve was not opening. A sound midway between a whistle and a sigh, "whhhhhooooo": the aortic valve was not closing.

We consulting doctors knew that Ms. Green had had a sore

throat two weeks before. We knew that it had been caused by a streptococcus infection, that she had been ill like this before, and that she had not taken the penicillin she knew she should. In short, we knew that she had rheumatic fever complicated by rheumatic heart disease. Most young American doctors had never seen a patient with this disease, which has nearly vanished from the United States but was still common in the Caribbean nation of her birth.

Mavis Green's personal doctor, a researcher, on a sort of sabbatical from his lab, had come to our staff to enhance his clinical skills. Though he studied this very disease, he had not personally cared for such a patient before. His laboratory had developed a new diagnostic test, so he first sent Ms. Green's blood specimen to his laboratory, then had asked us, the arthritis doctors, to consult.

Those of us who had previously seen patients with this disease were certain. "It *is* rheumatic fever," we said. "This girl is very sick. You had better start treatment at once." We thought it was urgent, so urgent that we did not wait. Normally we simply advise, but now we wrote a direct prescription in the physician's order book.

When we came back later, Ms. Green's condition was much worse. No, she told us between gasps, her treatment had not yet begun. Disbelieving, we checked the medication book. She was right. The treatment had not begun. We went back to the order book. Her doctor, we saw, had canceled our order after we had left the floor.

He came to the floor. "Why did you do this?" our senior doctor asked him in anger. "Why did you not treat this girl?"

"Because," Ms. Green's doctor replied, "my laboratory's test came back negative. She does not have rheumatic fever."

"Your test is wrong," the senior doctor shouted. "This lady

does have rheumatic fever. She needs treatment! She needed it yesterday! She needed it the day before yesterday! She needs it now! Get it started! Now!"

Ms. Green's doctor complied this time. He had no choice, because our senior doctor was the chairman of medicine at the hospital. As such he could overrule every doctor on the hospital staff. The research doctor also had no choice because even he could see that Ms. Green's status was now critical. Treatment began within the hour. She regained her health over the next few weeks.

Sometime later Ms. Green's doctor interrupted our weekly consultation rounds. His test had not been wrong, he wanted to say. His test had, indeed, confirmed that Mavis Green had rheumatic fever. Yet this did not contradict what he had told us before, he continued. His laboratory had reexamined the blood specimen, in fact, had done so several times. "Most of the time," he said, oblivious to the irony, "the result was positive."

I was speechless. To the scientist-physician, "most of the time," p less than 5 percent, was enough. A scientist's truth. Good enough for science, perhaps. Not good enough for clinical care.

A colleague suspected that a certain brain substance occurs only in lupus patients and, among them, only in those with a personality change called "lupus psychosis." (Lupus psychosis is not a real psychosis. It is more like delirium, and very disabling.) To confirm her hypothesis, my colleague needed to test many patients. I gave her blood samples from some of mine. She asked me to categorize each patient by means of a list I checked off and put in a sealed envelope. (This scientific method was correct: only I knew the diagnoses, and only she knew the test results. I could not bias her results, and she could not bias my classification.) Please tell me, she asked, whether each sample came from someone who does or does not have lupus psychosis.

It is not always easy to tell about this psychosis. Sometimes a patient's personality change is very subtle; sometimes drugs cause similar symptoms; sometimes patients are depressed because they are depressed. I answered my colleague accordingly: these patients do have lupus psychosis, these do not, and this group of patients (the largest), I'm not so sure about. When she opened the envelope, my colleague refused to accept my third category. Yes or no, she demanded, no in-betweens. I hemmed and hawed. This patient, I guessed, was 75 percent yes and 25 percent no. She took that to mean yes. For that one, 45 percent yes and 55 percent no, she wrote down no. Eventually she wore me down. I, unconvinced, said yes or no for each patient.

The brain substance, she concluded, does indicate who has lupus psychosis. It also tells us how lupus affects the brain. She published her study in a widely read medical journal. Others repeated and confirmed her result. As a definer of a medical truth, my colleague was right. Doctors now use her test to give a yes or no answer. But I know the patients on whom the test was first described, and I remain just a bit skeptical.

I also once helped describe a new laboratory test. A friend had shared with me a method to measure a new antibody. I used his test on pregnant lupus patients. The antibody, I found, identifies unborn babies likely to die. This conclusion has been confirmed many times. The antibody test is now widely used.

Less well known is that in my first paper I used a laboratory method that both my friend and I later found to be wrong. We corrected the flaws, and the test now works well. One reason why the wrong method gave us the right answer is funny—in retrospect. When I first worked on the test, I had not paid much attention to the temperature in the laboratory. It was summer, and our air-conditioning was erratic. The test worked correctly when the room was 72°F, but at higher temperatures, which happened when the air-conditioning failed, it gave a different result. By chance, the hot-day tests came out the right way. We eventually figured this out—after I had published my paper. When we corrected the test, I retested the specimens from my first paper. If the room temperature had been constant, I would not have come to the result I did. Yet in the last nine years, my original wrong paper has been cited in other printed articles 381 times.

Which is the greater truth? That the test does predict pregnancy problems? Or that my first paper was wrong? Truth is relative, not absolute. When there are hierarchies of truths, scientific "facts" are part of—but never the whole—argument.

Scientists use an inelegant maxim to deal with experimental results that intuitively seem wrong. If you see someone spit into the test tube, they say, it is permissible to discard the test. If you do not see someone spit into the test tube, you must include the result. In other words, all data count unless you can precisely and with certainty identify the experimental flaw. To assume that a(n unseen) flaw exists is bad science.

The spit-in-the-test-tube rule poses an interesting problem. Nonscientists assume—and scientists do not demur—that the results of most scientific experiments look like this:

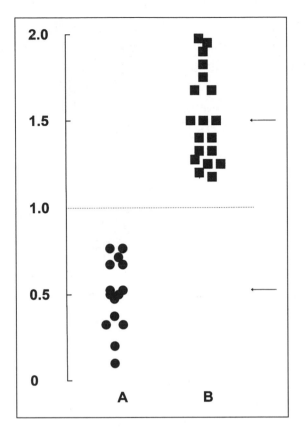

In this figure, the value 1 (with the line of dots) is the upper limit of normal. Samples (the circles and squares) represent a blood or other scientific test. Those which give results less than 1 (below the line) are normal, those greater than 1 (above the line) are abnormal. In a typical medical experiment, all the subjects in one group (A, the circles) are normal; subjects in the test group (B, the squares) are ill—patients with fever, sore throat, joint pain, and heart inflammation—in other words, people like Mavis Green suspected to have rheumatic heart disease. In this chart, everyone in group B has an abnormal test. The arrows point to the averages for each group.

People in group A average about 0.5 and those in group B about 1.5. Let us suppose the experiment is a blood test, a test like the one Mavis Green's doctor devised; in this example all the normals have a normal test (less than 1) and all the ill patients have an abnormal test (greater than 1). The results are clean. Do the test. The results will tell you who has the disease.

Would that it were so! Scientific data more often look like this:

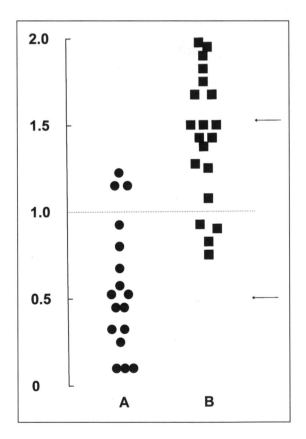

Here the average for group A is again about 0.5 and for group B again about 1.5. But this time there is an overlap between the groups. The results for the bottom six patients in group B and the top five patients in group A are about the same, between about 0.8 and 1.2, an indeterminate zone which is neither positive nor negative. Because the averages for the two groups have not changed, the test still says to a scientist that group A differs from group B. An honest scientist speaks of the overlap. But to condense data to the core, the textbooks will eventually include the averages, 0.5 and 1.5, and not the individual points, will mention positive and negative tests, saying something like this: "Patients with this disease have tests averaging 1.5, and normals have tests averaging 0.5." Users of the test will forget about the indeterminate zone. Uncritical scientists—and doctors—will still think the test unequivocally says yes or no.

The priority for science is: Does the test say that A is different from B? In the second chart, the answer for a scientist is yes. But medicine imposes a stricter priority: Is the test true each and every time it is run? Say it differently: Does the individual count? In the second chart, the answer for a doctor is that the test is correct "most of the time."

A more maddening circumstance is this one:

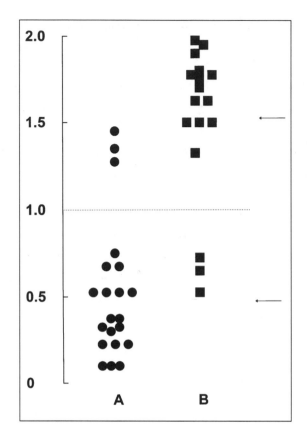

Here, most but not all of the subjects in group A, and most but not all in group B, behave in the expected way, very much as in the second chart. The averages are once again 0.5 for group A and 1.5 for group B. But this time three patients in group A and three in group B clearly differ from the rest. They are outliers. Invisible spit in the test tube? Perhaps the classification criteria are wrong (normality for group A; swollen joints, sore throat, scarred heart valves, fever, heart inflammation for group B). The top three samples in group A might be patients who have rheumatic fever without symptoms. The bottom three samples in group B might be patients who have symptoms like those of rheumatic fever but in fact suffer from a different disease. Or are the outliers a result of a chance event that closer analysis will identify? Maybe the test doesn't work on very hot days? Or a laboratory reagent has gone bad? Perhaps the test is inherently unstable. Or perhaps people vary more than laboratory animals do.

Scientists and doctors will read these data differently. For scientists, group A differs from B in all three graphs, and they can comfortably conclude that A does differ from B. If the scientist has done his work well, another scientist will do the same experiment and get the same result. But for the doctor, the test failed to classify eleven patients the second time, and incorrectly identified six patients in the third. The scientist wants to know that his data are statistically valid; the doctor wants to know that his patient will get well. Different priorities, and different truths.

Buried in the scientists' "truth" is uncertainty. Trap a scientist in a corner, talk to him one-on-one, poke a finger into his chest, and he will acknowledge ambiguity. In private, he may even admit that his categorical "yes" is often a "maybe yes" or a "mostly yes." But place that scientist face to face with a historian or sociologist or politician—or jury, or classroom, or doctor?—and you will hear him say, "Science is hard facts, verifiable facts. (Medicine is not.) Science represents absolute truth. (Medicine does not.) End of story."

Most doctors do not agree.

5

BUDGET CUTS

AN ANCIENT STAIN

There is a dark brown stain on Winnie Brown's medical chart, and the pages are warped. They were damaged a long time ago. The chart, wrinkled, curled, annoys me because it does not sit neatly in the stack of my afternoon's work. It makes the stack tilt and fall to the side.

I stare at the stain and my mind wanders. The stain is no Rorschach test. It is a Proustian moment. The stain and the warped paper take me back to the time when we doctors and our patients both knew about life in which social support systems failed.

Winnie Brown and I met in the wee hours of a snowy winter morning under dimmed nighttime hospital lights, while I examined this young, ill, and feverish woman, moaning softly, twisting and turning in bed, holding her head. The residents had called me in because they had diagnosed brain inflammation, Ms. Brown had a rash, and they thought the rash told them the reason she was ill; they wanted to begin treatment immediately. I was the senior physician. The rules were that I had to concur before they could start.

Ms. Brown's mother was at her side. Ms. Brown was a bank teller, she told me, who last worked two days before. The residents worried. Although the patient was awake and talking to them, she did not appear to think coherently enough to handle a job like that. When they asked her to perform simple arithmetical tasks she became confused. I asked her some additional questions. And I agreed: her thinking did not seem clear.

The residents had already drawn blood for laboratory tests. The critical results would not be available for several days. But her rash was the best clue we had. It told me instantly and unequivocally: lupus. The residents had been right. The confusion and incoherence had to be lupus brain inflammation. We started emergency treatment within minutes. By morning Ms. Brown was in deep coma. We were not surprised. The treatment, we knew, would take days, even weeks, to have effect. Her recovery—she did recover—was stormy and slow. It was weeks before she was fully conscious. It took more than a year before she could walk and talk normally again. Her health continued to be fragile for several years. She lost her job, of course, and with it her health insurance coverage. Our hospital social service department applied for Medicaid, then for a Social Security Disability allowance, on her behalf. These allowances supported her medical care and permitted her to stay in her home, to eat, and to travel to and from the clinic during the many months of her recovery.

Then Medicaid was cut back, briefly, in the early 1980s, as part of a general budget retrenchment. To doctors, the cutback resembled the warning at the time of the oil embargo of the mid-1970s that fossil fuel would one day run out. An oracle's voice cried: Pay attention! Here is what might be! But Medicaid is for the poor, and Social Security Disability is for those whose voices are weak, so the protest was unheard. Medicaid did not cease entirely, of course. Like the gasoline supplies, it became scarce, and only for a fairly short time. Eligibility criteria for Medicaid coverage tightened—a lot. In the gasoline crisis we saw a majority of our nation discomfited because they were unable to buy fuel. Everyone noticed, and the entire nation became very angry. In the Medicaid cutbacks a minority of the nation was unable to obtain medical care and almost no one took note.

Patients I had known for years abruptly lost their Medicaid support. The mechanism of termination was cruel. It did not require those patients to prove why they should remain covered. Instead, they were first removed from the rolls and then asked to prove (in person) why they should be reinstated—not an easy job if you depend on a wheelchair for transportation, do not speak English, have a mental disability, or are discouraged by long lines, churlish clerks, and constantly busy telephones. To get Medicaid coverage again, even those who had been disabled for years had to prove their eligibility anew. Many of my medically stable patients delayed their clinic appointments or stopped coming to see us altogether because they were physically and socially too weak to speak in their own defense. Some returned by ambulance when they ran out of medicine and became so ill that, in desperation, their families or the police brought them back to us, much sicker than they had ever been before. Despite the risk, that ploy worked, because it was easy to reinstate a patient hospitalized in an emergency to Medicaid.

Sometimes, to get patients back on the rolls, we doctors acted on our own. We overstated their symptoms if necessary to guarantee renewal of their eligibility. We invented reasons to hospitalize them so that we could give them the needed medication—why give a pill when an intravenous infusion will do just as well? Before the cutbacks, Medicaid had paid taxi fares to bring disabled persons to the clinic—a reasonable disbursement, since the disabilities usually prevented the patients from using subways or buses (which did not yet "kneel" for disabled riders). After the cutbacks, Medicaid paid only for ambulance calls. So when we needed to see a particular patient, we upgraded our description of the disability and ordered an ambulance. In the end it cost more, but at least we kept some patients in the treatment programs.

Like the stain on Winnie Brown's chart, the days when we lost Medicaid are dark and ugly. Ms. Brown had once had both a job and health insurance. Because of her illness she lost both. Social Security Disability had been her safety net—until the cutbacks. By the new rules, this young woman, still shy of her twentieth birthday, still needing a four-legged walker to prevent her from falling, and still speaking with the slurred, staccato speech that sounds like drunkenness to a layman but says diseased cerebellum to a doctor, was, according to the new Medicaid criteria, healthy enough to be on her own, no longer eligible for the support that gave her access to our clinic.

She and I disagreed with the new rule. We submitted a formal appeal for reinstatement, but we knew that even under the best circumstances the appeal process would take months. So, with the hospital administrators looking the other way, I cared for her, quasi-legally, as an unregistered, free patient in my private office rather than in the clinic, where she would have been charged what she could not afford to pay. I borrowed medications for her from other patients when I could and from a sympathetic pharmacist when I could not. When I needed to check her blood tests, I drew blood samples in my own office rather than send her to the hospital laboratory, which also would have charged her. I usually submitted these samples under false names and billed the costs to my research grants. (This was not completely immoral; I had some private grant money that had been donated for my discretionary use.) Sometimes friendly laboratory technicians did favors for me and ran the tests without recording them in the billing books. A few times I reached into my own pocket to pay for Ms. Brown's taxi and bus fares, and sometimes our social service department helped out from their own emergency funds. At one visit, washing her arm with an antiseptic, to draw a blood specimen, I spilled the antiseptic on her hospital chart. It stained the pages brown, and the paper warped.

I saw Ms. Brown frequently, often weekly, during that critical period. She is now well. Six years ago, when I moved from New York, I transferred her care to another physician, but she still calls me from time to time. She has a husband and a child and lives in the Bronx. Her son was one of the smallest surviving babies of my lupus pregnancy studies, just one and three-quarters pounds at birth. Not to worry: at age ten he won a countywide spelling bee.

Despite its gruesome beginning and its sociologically difficult middle part, Ms. Brown's medical history is a success story about lupus treatment. It is so good, in fact, that I used it to talk to Congress about how medical research saves lives. I made a big poster, three feet wide and four high, from a photograph I had taken of her, her husband, and her newborn son; I was particularly proud of her and her son at that time: I had just learned about the spelling bee.

Ms. Brown's days on Medicaid and on Social Security Disability are long since past. Still, there is the reminder on her chart, which neither she nor I need. For she remembers, and I remember, that vile period, when budget cutting briefly dismembered her safety net.

UTILIZATION COMMITTEES

When I was a child, my grandfather had his first heart attack. I remember it well, an imposing scene for a seven- or eight-year-old. The oxygen tent. My mother and grandmother crying quietly in the corner. My grandfather, pale, sweating, feeble. I was impressed that he was forbidden to shave himself, to his annoyance. Hospital barbers shaved heart-attack patients as they recovered. No physical exertion, not even shaving, was permitted them during the prescribed six-week period of absolute bed rest.

A decade and a half later, when I was a medical student, the rules for heart-attack patients had become more liberal. The magic number of weeks for bed rest was no longer six but three. Patients could get out of bed after the first week, but only into a "cardiac" chair, specially designed to put minimum strain on the heart.

Then we entered the modern world. The question "Why?" was asked more often. Why six weeks or why three? What would happen if patients got out of bed on the very first day? To answer the question new studies were done. It turned out that some heart-attack patients can walk and leave the hospital in just a few days. The same turned out to be true for patients having their hips replaced, or giving birth, or having their gallbladders removed. Traditional hospital stays, we doctors learned far too late, were, by habit rather than by considered thought, extravagant.

It would be nice to think that we doctors figured this all out on our own, but that is not true. Medicare had devised a system of payment criteria, called Diagnosis Related Groups, or DRGs, which assigned reimbursement for each of 495 diagnoses. Average lengths of stay across the country were calculated, then shaved a little. The calculation was more complex than that, but what Medicare paid the hospitals depended mostly on the number of hospital days allowed for any diagnosis. Each patient was allowed only one—a hospital could not be paid for both a heart attack and pneumonia in the same patient—though there was a small add-on for complex cases. The hospital then received the assigned amount as payment, regardless of what the real costs had been. Under the DRG system, a hospital able to discharge in four days a patient with a diagnosis rated at five days would be paid for the full five and would make a profit. If the patient stayed six days, whether because he had a temperature of 104 degrees or because a snowstorm had shut the city down, the hospital lost money. The DRG system was designed to reward efficiency. Responding, hospital Utilization Committees began to challenge doctors whose patients stayed around too long. Health maintenance organizations now push the challenges further.

Under such prodding we doctors (and patients) discovered, sometimes to our surprise, that the world did not collapse if carpal-tunnel and cataract surgery were done in outpatient clinics rather than on patients in hospitals, if coronary bypass patients got out of bed the first day after surgery, or if patients with infections received their intravenous antibiotic infusions at home. Such changes emptied our overcrowded hospitals. The Census Bureau tells us that in 1972 there were 142 hospital beds for every thousand persons in the population; in 1993, 119. In 1970, there were 1,122 hospital days for every thousand persons; this fell to 684 by 1994, and hospital occupancy fell from 78 to 68 percent. With excess bed capacity, hospitals converted some of their acute-care beds to halfway-house beds, nursing-home beds, or rehabilitation beds. Much money was saved.

Fewer hospital days mean less expensive health care, and most patients are better served than they were before. The bureaucratic name for this process is "utilization management." The transition to effective utilization management was not seamless, of course. Some newborns discharged on their first day in this world suffered missed diagnoses of preventable mental retardation—phenylketonuria (a treatable type of metabolic abnormality) or kernicterus (treatable jaundice)—because the tests done to exclude these diagnoses are inaccurate when done just after birth or were not done at all because the babies were not available for long enough. Some rapidly discharged surgery patients had to be rapidly readmitted with reopened or infected incisions. An occasional mother did not feel ready to return to her toddlers at home the very day she gave birth to her newest child. The missed diagnoses of newborns, and the concern of new mothers, led some states to pass laws—and the President in 1996 to sign a federal law—that required hospitals to provide at least forty-eight hours of care after delivery. This development itself is extraordinary. Government is writing the doctors' orders! Is government intervening in a relationship between a woman and her doctor, or is it protecting patients against the greed of a health-care payer? Your answer depends on which of two philosophies you hold: either government is the safety net for all of us or individual (including corporate) rights override our collective rights. My own response is that I trust government more than I do corporations, but prefer that the doctor and patient, together and unencumbered, decide the issue.

Here and there, a doctor or hospital administrator has noted that it is profitable if a patient dies on the first hospital day, costly to the hospital if, through vigorous action of its doctors, the patient recovers and is discharged after a long hospitalization. A quick death helps the hospital, since the patient's length of stay is less than that for which the DRG will pay. A patient's survival might harm it (stay longer than the DRG allows). Even thinking such thoughts suggests heinous scenarios, but I am not personally aware that anyone has actually encouraged death for a hospital's gain. Moreover, most patients are not harmed by the abbreviated stays. Hospital stays are efficient today. Much money is saved.

No hospital or HMO administrator earns his salary if he does not scan the computer printouts that cross his desk each day. These printouts tell him that Dr. Jones moves patients rapidly, that Dr. Jones's patients consistently earn a profit for the hospital. Dr. Smith's patients, on the other hand, always overstay their allowable DRG days, and Dr. Smith puts the hospital in the red. The administrator can choose among several explanations and actions.

The easiest explanation is the first one. One logical remedy is to ask Dr. Smith to undergo training in efficient patient care, another is to fire him. A second explanation is that Dr. Smith sees sicker or older patients than Dr. Jones does, or, conversely, that Dr. Jones "cherry-picks" patients who are likely to be inexpensive and refuses patients who are likely to be costly. Is Dr. Jones immoral or unprofessional? I doubt the hospital much cares. A third explanation is that Dr. Smith's patients are older, perhaps mostly in their seventies, while Dr. Jones's are in their forties. (This is not an unusual scenario, since doctors' practices tend to age with them.) A fourth is that Dr. Smith may be known for taking on the most difficult and most complex cases. The patients may be costly, but his fame brings business to the hospital; the less experienced, or less courageous, Dr. Jones may choose the simple cases Dr. Smith is too busy to see; the entire patient recruitment might still lead to a net profit for the hospital; and Dr. Smith may be more valuable to the hospital than he seems. Another explanation is that, compared with Dr. Smith, Dr. Jones takes too many chances, does not do enough tests, discharges pa-

Dr. Smith	Dr. Jones
is less efficient	is very efficient
sees sicker than average patients	avoids sick patients
has a practice with many old people	avoids old people
is referred the hardest cases	cherry-picks his patients
is too cautious	is reckless

tients too early. Or, conversely, that Dr. Smith is too cautious, does too many tests, does not discharge patients early enough.

A final explanation is that Dr. Jones and Dr. Smith are basically similar, and statistical artifacts have made the difference: perhaps one extremely out-of-range patient favorably skewed Dr. Jones's average or unfavorably skewed Dr. Smith's. Explaining the difference between a Dr. Jones and a Dr. Smith is not simple.

I have had some experience with this issue. To "help" us "evaluate" our own practices, my hospital sent us physicians a monthly accounting of our patients, pointing out whether their hospital stays were above or below the DRG average. In theory, it was an educational effort: if your patients' stays are high, learn from your colleagues what you are doing wrong. But we all read it as: if you keep costing us money, we won't be able to keep you on our staff. This occurred in the era before HMOs. With HMOs, "education" is no longer the aim.

There is clearly a threat here, but it is not, as you may have

thought, merely a threat to doctors. The threat is to patients
who are very ill. The message to doctors is: avoid sick patients.
The larger threat to the great hospitals is: if you pride yourself
on caring for the most difficult patients or on hiring the doctors who accept the hardest challenges, you may soon be bank-
rupt. Better to cherry-pick and stay solvent. That is a worthy
aim, to be sure, but if accountants have the final word, hospitals will avoid the tough cases. You may think this makes
good economic sense, but what if the tough case is you?

I know the effect of this threat well. I saw it face-on in my
colleagues when I left New York. After twenty years, I had been
pleased with the medical practice I had built. My practice included the most severe cases of rheumatic diseases, ones over
which other doctors had thrown up their hands. I used to joke
with the intensive-care unit staff that at least two, sometimes
four, of their beds had my name written on them, for my
patients always occupied them. The ICU staff liked them, because they were mostly young, and they usually survived.

Now, as I left for Washington, I had to find new doctors for
my patients. I assumed, naïvely it turns out, that my younger
colleagues would take them willingly. One by one my colleagues offered excuses. One said, "Please give me just your
interesting patients, so long as they are not too sick." Another
said, "Your patients take too much time. I can't move them
in and out fast enough." In the end only the threat that I
would refer my patients to a rival hospital across town forced
some of my colleagues to say yes.

This all occurred at the very beginning of "utilization management," before HMOs began seriously to fire doctors whose
patients cost too much. But I know that the cost of medical
care in the United States is rising rapidly. And it may be that
we will choose to ration hospital beds on the basis of severity
of disease, adopt a sort of survival-of-the-fittest philosophy,

practice triage as on a battlefield, abandon those whose illnesses cost too much. In the future, very sick people may not
be able to get care.

To penalize doctors who care for very sick patients, claiming
that inefficiencies and not the patients' needs account for the
costs, will make physicians the enemies of their patients. Imagine a doctor whose first thought, as you walk through the door,
is: Is this patient going to be a profit or a loss? Partnership
and mutual trust are bound to be destroyed. To have a doctor
assess your illness and think: If I care for this person I will lose
my job, is to destroy everything a patient expects of medicine.
It mocks every moral value in a physician's creed.

Alice Tsang arrived at our hospital by a traditional route: a
small community hospital saw that it did not have the facilities
to deal with the cataclysm her very complex illness posed, and
that they were losing this patient. "Train wreck coming in,"
we learned, either from her husband or from her local physician, I don't remember. And so we waited in the emergency
room for the transport ambulance and for our first look at this
woman. She was, we were told, ravaged by convulsions, antibodies were destroying her blood cells at a rate faster than they
could be replaced, her kidneys were not working at all, and
one heart valve was destroyed by infection.

The ambulance arrived. She was worse than we had been
told. No question where she belonged: within minutes she was
in our intensive-care unit, and she did not leave it for three
months.

Patients as ill as Alice Tsang seldom survive. Death often
occurs when one critical organ system fails, and Ms. Tsang had
several systems—heart, kidney, blood, brain—failing at once.
A former student of mine, in his first rotation as a medical

resident, fairly whimpered as he spoke: "You told me all these diseases could happen," he said, "but you never said they could all happen to the same person at the same time!"

I have no idea what Ms. Tsang's hospitalization cost. It was certainly tens and possibly hundreds of thousands of dollars. But fifteen years later she is well, takes no medications, comes once a year for her annual checkup, and is a successful lawyer in New Jersey. (She handled malpractice law before she fell ill, and it amuses me to tell her that her returning to her practice is proof that she did not have full brain recovery.) She raises Dalmatian dogs, a particularly touching point for me, since I grew up with three. She sends me Christmas cards with pictures of these dogs. Tells me their names, too, but I never remember them.

When the New Jersey hospital first made contact with us, they knew we would take in Ms. Tsang, and our hospital knew I would accept a very sick patient with her diagnosis. For my part, accepting that challenge was why I became a doctor. Though Ms. Tsang's hospitalization lasted months, no one complained. These events took place before Utilization Committees were born. There were no DRG rules telling us that her illness allowed only eight hospital days. And her insurance paid the full bill.

Muriel Taylor's hospitalization also lasted for months, but she fell critically ill after Utilization Committees rather than before.

Strong-willed, religious, considerate, Mrs. Taylor was crippled by rheumatoid arthritis, which had destroyed most of her joints. Arthritis was only one of her problems. She was nearly blind. She had had a couple of heart attacks, and her blood pressure was much too high. Neither her lungs nor her thyroid gland worked very well. I thought she was unlucky to have so many different afflictions. She disagreed, because not one of them had truly slowed her down. With the help of close friends from her church, she lived by herself and vigorously contributed to her community.

At one point arthritis damaged her wrist so that she could no longer use her hand. We did a surgical repair. After the surgery—actually, as she was waiting in the lobby for her ride home—she felt chest pain. It was a new heart attack. We immediately readmitted her to the hospital (it was too soon after her discharge—a black mark for me), and she did not do well. Her lungs filled with fluid; she developed blood clots; her intestines twisted (necessitating abdominal surgery, a colostomy, repeat surgery, closure of the colostomy), and she had blood clots again. Three ICU admissions, two abdominal surgeries, and eight months later, we finally sent her back home, again well, fully alert, and as able to participate in her community as she had before. We sent a visiting nurse to check on her every day for a while, then each week, then each month. She stayed in this state (well for her) for another five years, until her heart deteriorated and she died, peacefully, rapidly, and without pain.

None of the catastrophes that happened to Mrs. Taylor during those eight months stopped me from getting twice-weekly notes from my department chairman reminding me that my patient had overstayed, then very much overstayed, then very, very much overstayed the time the DRGs allotted for her diagnosis. In the DRG lexicon, heart attack was the only diagnosis we were allowed to list. We gained a couple of extra days for the second diagnosis, "complication or age over 65" (either one, no extra days for both), and no extra days for volvulus (twice, with eventual colostomy and colostomy repair), pulmonary infarction, atrial flutter, blindness, hypertension, rheumatoid arthritis, or nontoxic goiter. No one told me exactly what I should do, however, with a seventy-year-old, blind, crippled woman, rigged up to oxygen and to feeding and drainage tubes, yet fully alert, cheerful, and involved. I wasn't fired because of this lengthy hospitalization, of course. We hadn't reached that level of economizing—yet. But I got the point, more or less, and so did my colleagues. That is why they did not want to accept my patients.

Being an optimist of the Anne Frank stamp—believing, that is, in the essential goodness of man—I do not think that it was greed for faster "throughput" that made my colleagues respond the way they did. Nor do I think it was unwillingness to assume hard challenges. Rather, I think they saw more clearly than I did what the future held: if you continue to encourage very sick patients to come here, the chairman's notes to me had said, you risk your hospital appointment, hence your job.

Here is a puzzle: If elite institutions, whose reputations rely on their great expertise, shun the sickest patients, are they still elite? What added value do the great hospitals offer if not the ability to do a better job than anyone else? They have always sharpened their skills by taking the sickest patients. If they avoid these patients, their skills will weaken and disappear, and the elite hospitals will exist no more.

Should we, to save money, exclude from care those persons unlucky enough to have complex diseases? Should we ration by luck of the draw? If you have a cheap diagnosis, come to us. Appendicitis? No problem. Carcinoid tumor of the appendix? Too expensive; go elsewhere, if you can find someone to take you. Should we refuse patients the right to consult experts? "Well, no," says the Hometown, U.S.A., HMO doctor, "I've never seen a case of Wegener's granulomatosis before, but they don't want you at the university hospital, and I'll be criticized if I refer you elsewhere, so you stay with me. We'll muddle through." Is this the way it will be?

We can establish, and subsidize, centers of medical excellence for difficult patients. We don't even have to start them from scratch. They already exist as our university hospitals and specialty clinics. The problem is that, because they are paid on the same scale as community hospitals (which have the luxury of avoiding the very sick patients), they cannot compete very well, and are tempted to avoid very sick patients, too. The game is to duck the ball. The patient is the bouncing ball. Everybody loses.

There are not so many very sick patients that caring for them puts the national health-care bill at risk. If we maintain medical centers of excellence for very sick patients, there will be inconveniences, to be sure. Some patients will have to travel long distances. But that is not new—it is how Alice Tsang came to our emergency room. The elite centers must be paid extra for the care they give the very ill, or they will be at financial risk, and there will be no recourse for the patients. There may be better options that I do not have the vision to see. But so long as the Alice Tsangs and the Muriel Taylors are not abandoned, any workable option is okay.

HMOs

I saved a life once—well, actually, more than once. I'm not talking about the more or less mechanical operations doctors do by rote: cardiopulmonary resuscitation, finding a tumor early enough to do something useful, administering a drug to stop a chaotic heart rhythm. That type of lifesaving can be done when one knows a few basic, not very abstruse, facts and applies them quickly when necessary. Although one gets an adrenaline charge from these, one's intellect is not fully engaged. I'm also not talking about making an obscure diagnosis, searching through medical journals, finding the right researcher with the right test, using every bit of mental power one can muster. That type of lifesaving is also stimulating, but very much a matter of luck—what one has read recently, what specific little detail triggers the right recall of the right journal article. It is pleasant to feel brilliant for a few minutes, but it does not signify an accomplishment that calls on a lifetime of accrued talents. It does not simultaneously test all your skills and prove that the accumulated trivia of your medical work have been collected with a purpose and are not just detritus clogging your brain. Making a brilliant diagnosis may in any case not save the life at hand. The disease may not be lethal. There may be no treatment. Chronic-disease doctors are not trauma surgeons. They do not usually work in intensive-care wards. They do not deal daily with emergency life-and-death decisions, though long-term life-and-death decisions, yes, and quality-of-life decisions most certainly. But for us, the moments when all one's accumulated experience pulls together and enables one to make the correct decision within minutes are fairly rare.

The time I saved a life was one of those instants. For a few moments I had to use all my skills: of knowledge, of experience, and of intuition. I had to have close personal knowledge of the patient and a thorough understanding of her illness, of course. I also needed an instinct to know that what was before my eyes was not ordinary, that I needed to look harder. For me, that experience is what being a doctor is all about. On the other hand (to my mind) if you cannot react correctly, you're not really a doctor at all.

What happened was rather simple. All I did was respond to a telephone call, make a quick examination, and make another call. The patient's family and other doctors did most of the real work. But if I had temporized or not responded instinctively, the patient would have died. The whole thing was so instinctive, in fact, that there's not much of a story to tell.

I had known Brenda O'Neill for several years. Before I met her, a routine blood test had shown low blood platelets, which causes a risk of bleeding. The low-platelet count had caused her no problem—it worried the doctors more than it did her. I saw her only because she had lost two pregnancies. I was doing research on the antibody, an abnormal protein, in her blood that was causing the pregnancies to fail. Brenda and Jeff O'Neill wanted to try pregnancy again.

My research was not very helpful to them; she lost two more pregnancies under my care. Still, as I worked with her, I came to know her and her family well. And several months before the lifesaving time, I had a long discussion about her future with her and her parents. I had explained why I was pessimistic about a new pregnancy, though otherwise I thought her long-term prognosis was rather good.

I was wrong.

Brenda and Jeff were vacationing with her parents on a resort island in New England, five or six hours' drive plus a ferry ride away from home. I don't remember why I knew they were there. Probably she had mentioned the trip in a conversation we had had, or maybe she had asked me to fill a prescription beforehand. She called from the island. Brenda had developed what seemed to be a flu or a cold. She had gone to a local physician. He had prescribed an antibiotic. She wanted to know if it was okay to take it. I was glad she had called. I like to have that type of relationship with my patients. They are in charge of their own health but cautious enough to double-check when a new doctor enters the scene. Mrs. O'Neill and I had once had a chat about what to do if you get sick while traveling, and I had repeated my mantra: "A phone call is cheaper than a catastrophe."

The antibiotic was okay, I said. Her symptoms sounded non-descript. "Keep me informed," I offered. "Call again if the symptoms change."

The second call a day or so later was more troubling. Brenda still had a low-grade fever and still felt unwell. The local phy-sician wanted to admit her to their small hospital. I listened to the story, spoke to the doctor, and concurred. I had no specific thoughts, certainly no brilliant insight, and no expla-nation for my unease. I advanced my alert system. "Keep me informed," I told the O'Neills once again. "If you don't call me, I'll call you. What are your telephone numbers?" I get nervous when my patients, particularly those who do not fit textbook cases, are ill and in strange hands. The circumstances were good, though: the local physician was easy to talk to, accessible, and well informed; and the essential communica-tion lines were open.

The next day, Brenda did not look good, they said. Her parents were worried, and the local doctor was also worried. Nothing much to go on, but they all, including the doctor, repeated, "The local hospital is very small."

On the first day of medical school, our dean gave to each member of my class a copy of Sir William Osler's essay *Ae-quanimitas*, equanimity. You are now a doctor, Osler says in it. When you walk into a sickroom, people look to you. If you stay calm, they stay calm. If you don't, everyone will panic. Your equanimity is an important part of the cure.

As I listened on the telephone, I understood that *aequa-nimitas* had vanished from that small hospital on that small island off the New England shore. The family and I talked about whether Mrs. O'Neill could get to New York or whether she should go to Boston, with its large hospitals, at which I had friends. They said they'd like to come home. They could charter an airplane and bring her immediately. Okay, I said, while I arranged for a hospital bed.

The bed was not ready when they arrived, so I met the family at the hospital's front door. I was alarmed at what I saw. Nothing specific, but Mrs. O'Neill was not as alert as I would have wanted—more than just fatigue—and a number of things about her demeanor troubled me. My instinct told me that she was very ill. Her fever was not high, her laboratory tests were not seriously abnormal, but there were slight signs of infection in her blood, and her liver was just a little tender.

This is where the experience part comes in. Because I was discomfited, not by clear findings but by a hunch, I called a surgeon friend of mine. He came at once. Usually surgeons tell the medical doctors they want to operate. Usually the medical doctors argue no, but I reversed the order. I told the surgeon I wanted surgery as soon as possible. He, too, was puzzled by Mrs. O'Neill's condition, but we had worked together before; he knew my experience as I knew his. Within an hour Ms. O'Neill was in surgery. We found that her liver had ruptured because some of its arteries had clotted, and whole sections of the organ had been killed. That condition is very rare. Arteries supplying other major organs had also clotted. Her kidneys and heart were threatened, too. I had never seen anything like it before.

Within a few hours Mrs. O'Neill's kidneys failed totally. Then her heart failed partially. Her body filled with fluid. We treated her with every medicine we had. We washed her blood. We instituted dialysis to control the fluid and to extract the poisons her kidneys could no longer remove. Her liver did not work, so her skin turned yellow. Her heartbeat became erratic. Her lungs repeatedly filled with fluid, though we were able to reverse the deterioration each time. Over the next several days, with several setbacks, she began to rally. The heart strengthened, the lungs cleared, and her skin regained its normal color. Only the kidneys did not improve. The next weeks were difficult. We were able to discharge her from the hospital after two months, on dialysis for kidney failure, taking a pharmacyful of drugs. A year and a half later her kidneys revived. She discontinued dialysis and most of the medications, and was once again well. Several years have passed. She and Jeff now have two wonderful children. She lives a full life, like any young mother.

A few years after Mrs. O'Neill's crisis, and after I had seen a few more patients like her, I and my colleagues wrote a paper about her crisis. (Her condition had not been described in medical books before.) I gave lectures about it and learned that other doctors had seen it in patients of their own and not known what to call it or what to do. Of late, more papers about the syndrome have appeared. I now know that what happened is a rare, devastating complication of the abnormal antibody that Mrs. O'Neill carries. The syndrome is in the textbooks now.

Most patients with this syndrome die. Only a few patients, treated immediately and maximally, survive. Mrs. O'Neill was the first patient with the syndrome I ever saw and one of the very few who have lived. There had been no guidelines for me to follow. My knowing both her and her disease well enough to decide, on the basis of a tentative telephone call—instinct and experience—and, importantly, a favorable look from Above, saved her life.

The point of the story is not that I did something right, which I did, nor that even chronic-disease doctors have occasional dramatic moments, which they do. To understand my point, focus your attention on the timing, the sequence, and the geography of those critical forty-eight or seventy-two hours. Think about what might have happened if these events had occurred in the present day, if Mrs. O'Neill had belonged to an HMO.

Mrs. O'Neill fell ill in New England, not in New York. Under the rules today, she might have had to seek her insurer's permission to see the local physician, an inconvenience and a delay, perhaps enough of a deterrent to have prevented her first call. Her symptoms were quite vague. Permission might have been refused. She certainly would have had to seek permission from her insurer to be hospitalized and later transferred to New York. Once transferred, she would have had to go to her primary-care gatekeeper, not the specialist she knew (me). The gatekeeper would have had to get permission to call me in. I would have had to get permission from the HMO to hospitalize her for what seemed to be a flu but, to my instinct, just did not look right. Instinct that one cannot well articulate, that fits no diagnostic box, does not justify hospitalization if you belong to an HMO. The critical difference—which I would not have been able to explain to the HMO—is that I had known Brenda O'Neill for years, knew her well enough to intuit an imminent catastrophe, even though I could not put a label on what it was. (The doctor on the island had the same instinct. Because he knew neither her nor her disease well, he lacked *aequanimitas*. That I did know both gave me the confidence I needed to act.)

When a doctor calls an HMO to get authorization, he does not get an experienced physician on the line. The HMO asks the doctor to describe specific symptoms and to assign a specific diagnosis in advance. A clerk searches a computer screen and gives a reply. The doctor also gives the clerk a specific plan of action and projects the required number of hospital days, often further explaining why this patient cannot be cared for at home. Clearly I—and certainly not the gatekeeper physician—could not have sought these permissions or given clear answers in that very short time, by telephone, about a patient many hours away. I could have lied, of course, adding a symptom here, exaggerating one there, to get the authorization I wanted, but I am uncomfortable with dishonesty. I use it only when there is no other way.

If I had been an HMO physician, I would have had to get permission to call the surgeon, and the surgeon would have had to get permission to operate. I might not have had a choice of surgeons, might not have even met the assigned one before, much less have worked with him in the past. Had I or the surgeon not received permission or, worse, not have wasted time calling the (generally busy) HMO phone lines, we still would have donè what we did do, because that is the way we are. Likely the HMO would have refused to pay. That would have cost the hospital heavily. I would have risked a reprimand, if not a discharge. For Mrs. O'Neill, we used top-of-the-line experimental treatments on an emergency basis, and these treatments would certainly have been disallowed. HMOs cannot afford to pay for experimental treatments, because, according to Dr. Malik Hasan, the CEO of a large organization in California, cited in a *Time* article in January 1996, HMOs do function in "a Darwinian world."

It does not have to be that way. Payment decisions do not have to be made case by case. General principles can apply, freeing doctors to make patient-specific judgments. There can be national, not corporate, standards, and general guidelines. A clerk reading from a checklist should not tell a doctor how to treat his patient. Give the guidelines to the doctors, let them decide when which rule should apply. Review their decisions later, when the crises have passed. If the doctors were wrong, apply sanctions. But do not hobble emergency care.

The alternative for Mrs. O'Neill would have been to concede

that any one of the emergency decisions—by the local physician, the hospitalization in Massachusetts, the transfer to specialty care in New York, the surgical consultation, and the surgery itself—could or should have been denied. But to deny those decisions is to conclude that Mrs. O'Neill's life has no value in and of itself, saying that she is just one individual in a vast population of persons in the HMO, and if it looks as if she has an expensive illness, she should please die, for then the HMO will save money, and one death will not bias the statistics this year. I am not overstating the case. According to one HMO medical director's point of view (Dr. Sam Ho, cited in that same *Time* article of January 1996), fiduciary responsibility—not just to stay in business, but to produce comfortable profits—outweighs all else.

The argument is reasonable—to some. But doctors in practice work not with aggregate populations but with individual patients. They make individual decisions, often with families, mostly with patients. Brenda O'Neill made her own decisions during her entire crisis. I could not have been an apologist for, or the protector of, a system that would elect not to treat her because of the cost. Nor could I have acceded to a disembodied telephone voice that contradicted what, at the bedside, my clinician's heart knew to be right.

6

SPEAKING AS A NATION

"COMMON, CHRONIC, COSTLY, CRIPPLING"

In room 2358, on the second floor of the Rayburn House Office Building, the witnesses' table is twenty, maybe twenty-five feet long, and about three feet deep. It has a dark leather top. Eight chairs, tight together, line one side. Seated in one of them, I had little elbowroom. I am in the left center chair, facing the podium. My flip cards, neatly packaged in a leather folder, are before me. Four of my senior staff associates occupy the chairs to my left and one to my right. Each of them has a loose-leaf briefing book, four inches thick, with many pages dog-eared and color-coded, so that its bearer can quickly thrust in front of me the right answers to any question that we have predicted in our preparation sessions, and now hope may come. To my far left, at the end of the table, sit others of my staff, alert to place our posters on the easel they hold ready. The director of the National Institutes of Health (NIH) is two seats to my right, the deputy director next to him, and the Department of Health and Human Services representative is on her right. Ostensibly, they are there to back me up, but, if the truth be known, they are there to set the record straight— and pillory me later—if I say something that contradicts President Clinton's policy. My role, as director of one of NIH's institutes, is to ask Congress to appropriate funds for medical research.

In room 2358 of the Rayburn Building, old oil paintings on the walls add dignity and substance. There is a special clock high on the back wall, which those on the podium can see. Below the clock, unlabeled lights and buzzers transmit messages, the meanings of which I do not know, to announce the status of votes on the floor of the House of Representatives. When a buzzer sounds, the members of Congress abruptly leave their podium seats without so much as a by-your-leave, and vanish for a half hour or so to cast their votes. The witness waits at the table for their return.

Before me, on the podium, will soon sit my questioners, members of the Labor, Health and Human Services, and Education Subcommittee of the House of Representatives' Committee on Appropriations. Their table is grand, substantial, of dark hardwood, curving in a broad concave arc toward me. Democrats will sit on my left, Republicans on my right. Their chairs, high-backed, with arms, are covered in supple leather. My chair is less accommodating. I notice the contrast in comfort. Flags flank the table. The committee's seal is displayed high above.

Behind me are three rows of chairs spaced too close to give legroom. The chairs are occupied by people who have come to hear the testimony but who will not speak. Others stand in back and along the sides of the room. Many people have an interest in what I am about to say.

The entrance lobby and the hallways of the Rayburn Building are marble, and the halls themselves are broad, the ceiling very high. The oak doors are elegantly carved. Inside the hearing room, nearly floor-to-ceiling windows, facing north, open on but do not admit the bright sun. The windows cover most of the left wall. By necessity, my team has assembled very early. It is a lovely spring day.

Waiting, I gaze at the lawn outside.

Springtime in Washington is symphonic in scope and scale.

In Washington, spring's symphony starts in February, when the dreary winter cabbages (cabbages!), maroon anodyne for winter's brown and gray, rot and slowly disappear. The ornamental cabbages are only noise, a warm-up, for the orchestra preparing to play. The symphony begins in March: a few introductory notes, light, clear—daffodils, jonquils, and forsythia like strings and woodwinds, the clarinet in A. Tulips follow, red and white, lush hues. In early April there are small-bloom cherries, delicate, pink and white. Plum and peach trees flower. Then come more woodwinds and muted brass: full-flower cherries and apples, with their more intense reds; violet redbud; and tumescent magnolia, all crimson and purple and robust. The tempo rises to allegro. Deep, rich copper, the Japanese maples open their leaves—bassoons. White dogwood, then pink dogwood, spread their branches wide. In late April the whole orchestra joins in carmine display—percussion and brass and woodwind and strings and chorus, full voice, vivace, crescendo, Washington florissant, as, from their low places in the shadows, quietly, just a few buds at first, then suddenly ascendant, explosive, seeking the sun—white, rose, cherry, fuchsia, magenta, crimson, scarlet!—the azaleas reign.

I used to collect phrases of affirmation to energize me when I was low. Valéry's great poem "Le Cimitière marin," was one: "Stand tall in the new age! . . . A breeze—the sea's breath—

gives me back my soul . . . One must live!" And Thoreau's line "Walden was dead and is alive again" was another. To me, Washington's springtime is like those passages. It stimulates, invigorates, gives back the soul. Washington's springtime is the full chorus at the end of *The Marriage of Figaro*. "Everyone celebrate! *Corriam tutti a festeggiar!*"

In the hearing room in the Rayburn Building, I focused my thoughts back to the business of the day. The subcommittee's chairman entered and took his seat. The room hushed. He opened the meeting. I adjusted the microphone before me.

"Four words that start with the letter *c*," I began, "convey what I want to say. I am going to talk about diseases that are *common*, about diseases that are *chronic*, about diseases that are *costly*, and about diseases that are *crippling*."

My purpose that day was narrow. I needed to make clear, in the seven minutes allowed for my opening statement, and in my replies to the questions that would follow, that rheumatic, orthopedic, dermatologic diseases affect many Americans—back pain, skin rashes, arthritis: they are *common*. That they cost the country $133 billion per year: *costly*. That they last lifetimes: *chronic*. And that they are very disabling: *crippling*.

I did not, that day, expand my comments to cover all human disease. I did not mention the politics of health care or the manner of its delivery. But in a different situation I might have, because the point would have been the same. After all, *cost* is at the very heart of our medical-care crisis. The cost of medical care comes from care for *common* diseases—arthritis, for instance, and osteoporosis. The research for which I that day sought money has as its aim making these illnesses less common. It will not do so in the short term, nor will it decrease the nation's burden of *chronic* illness, unless we very quickly and simultaneously find cures for many ailments: diabetes, high blood pressure, osteoporosis, arthritis, heart disease, stroke, Alzheimer's, bowel and bladder disease, skin disease, and all the cancers. Can we reduce *crippling*, then? Eventually, yes, but not likely very soon. Infirmity, nursing homes, walking and hearing and visual aids will stay with us for the near term.

High cost is here now and will remain. To solve a fiscal crisis, fiscal tools—reassignment of resources, priority setting, squeezing someone (doctors or patients or both)—are required. The prognosis for the health of our medical-care system is uncertain. The prognosis, as doctors say, is guarded. Used this way, the word is a euphemism—it means "not good." It means "poor."

The dollars we spend now, the dollars that create the fiscal crisis, mitigate the suffering of, and lessen the burden for, but do not now cure, persons whose illnesses are . . . common, chronic, costly, and crippling. Is the prognosis for their future guarded?

STOPPING EPIDEMICS

In late 1989 an epidemic of severe muscle pain, skin rashes, and unusual blood counts struck almost two thousand Americans. The victims had a common trait: they had used a "health food" product called L-tryptophan. Many victims died. Others were permanently crippled.

L-tryptophan is an amino acid, the left-hand (L) version of one of sixteen vital dietary amino acids. Almost any protein supplies the body with its tryptophan needs. Tryptophan forms a chemical, serotonin, which affects one's mood. An L-tryptophan supplement has been available in health-food stores for many years. For most of those years only a few psychiatrists and natural-health-food advocates knew it was for sale. But in the late 1980s L-tryptophan became a faddish non-prescription remedy for insomnia and depression. To meet the rising demand, its major manufacturer, a reputable pharmaceutical firm, changed the way it made the drug. Soon the cases of this new disease, the "eosinophilia-myalgia" syndrome, began to appear. (The manufacturer was not American. Because the product was classified as a food supplement, not a medicine, it had not been subject to regulation. Had it been classified as a drug or manufactured in America, the change in the manufacturing process would have been monitored and possibly the epidemic prevented.)

Within weeks the link between the epidemic and the new formulation of L-tryptophan was clear. The changed manufacturing process had apparently caused an undetected contamination. The Food and Drug Administration (FDA) immediately removed L-tryptophan from store shelves. The epidemic ended as abruptly as it had begun.

Stopping dramatic epidemics is now the stuff of popular fiction. Books and movies dwell on pandemics that are transported around the world in the time of an airplane flight. In the novels, throngs of doctors rush to the scene, race to their laboratories, and beseech grumpy, uncooperative, bureaucratic officials for resources. They usually solve the problem and save humanity.

It is not all fiction. There are true stories like this, too. The most impressive part of the stories, however, not often noted, is that there are doctors who can throng, rush, race, beseech, solve, and save. Where do the doctors throng from? And when they beg for resources, whom do they beg? Without a thronging-from place and a resource base, there would be no story. The epidemics might not stop.

The identification, the tracking, the risk defining, the research, and the preventive action all come from government science. The thronging-from place and the resource base are part of our national health-care budget. The United States government maintains research laboratories in Maryland, Georgia, Colorado, and many other places. The job of these laboratories is to keep scientific minds and technology and resources at their peak. The laboratories provide the people and technology to stop pandemics before they occur. They and the system are not perfect, of course. Sometimes they give false alarms—government scientists predicted a severe influenza epidemic in 1975–76, which did not occur—but despite such embarrassments, the success rate of the government laboratories is very high.

Government protects our health in many ways. Consider the early history of AIDS. When AIDS emerged in the 1980s, it appeared to be lethal. There was confusion and panic. It is really a new disease? Whom does it affect? Is it a gay disease? A Haitian disease? A disease of hemophiliacs? A drug addicts' disease? Is it one or several diseases? What are the common factors? How does it spread? Within a few years all these questions had been answered. A virus was found. Some treatments are now available, and in the future there may be vaccines. The recognition, tracking, risk defining, virus discovery, and treatment development occurred because government resources were there.

Government laboratories help to protect us from chronic illness. Some of them work on cancer, others on arthritis, heart disease, diabetes, Alzheimer's, osteoporosis, and a host of other ills—schizophrenia, drug addiction, birth defects, and environmental diseases. The work the government laboratories do is mostly *proactive*: they initiate and conduct new research on illnesses that affect us even when there is no public alarm. The *reactive* part—a possible new disease to identify and conquer—is important, but the reactive response relies on having technology and personnel *already in place*. Most "basic" medical research in this country is done either by government employees or by people paid by government grants. The immediate use of all government-supported research may not be immediately apparent, but that research is the foundation for treatments that will follow.

How does the system work? Here is an example of how government, using both its regulatory and its research powers, responded to a new problem.

I have earlier mentioned that rheumatologists called to public attention the unusual number of scleroderma patients who had had silicone breast devices implanted. The diagnosis was not in question. Scleroderma is rare and dramatic: the skin tightens and hardens; the patient's appearance changes. To see many patients in a single practice is unusual. To see many who had had breast implants as well sounded an alarm.

It is important to note that practicing doctors, seeing patients, first raised this alarm. Clinical observations like theirs produce only suspicions, but the public-health implications can be immense. Clinical observations are red flags. It was practicing doctors who pointed out a handful of brain degeneration cases in England in 1996 of what the world now knows of as "mad cow disease." Clinicians talked about a few young gay men with strange infections two decades ago—and it was AIDS. Individual practicing doctors first called attention to what we now call Legionnaires' disease, Lyme disease, Hanta virus, and other epidemics.

When the doctors' new reports suggested that implants might cause scleroderma, the FDA took charge. It quickly discovered that manufacturers of the implants had never questioned the long-term safety of the product. In other words, the FDA had no information it could use to reassure the public. While waiting for results from new (government-sponsored) studies, it had to choose between two unpleasant options: to frighten but protect the public by banning the devices (and risk opprobrium if new research proved they were harmless) or put more women at risk by staying silent (if the warnings about scleroderma were correct). The FDA chose the former option.

Whether the FDA made the right decision is not my point here. My point is that government agencies acted quickly on the public's behalf and that government-supported doctors did and continue to do the defining studies. The doctors that thronged, the resources they garnered, are as much part of the government's investment as its payment of Medicare bills.

COST-EFFECTIVENESS

Present wisdom says that Americans need and deserve to make intelligent, cost-effective, consumer-type choices about medical care. Health is a consumer good; it can be priced. Using the same techniques that we employ when we choose between a Mercedes-Benz SL 600 ($127,000) and a Mazda Miata ($26,000), both two-seat sports cars, luxurious but expensive versus functional and low-cost, we should choose among health-care plans. And why not use cost as a criterion? After all, what is the real difference in cars? Both the SL 600 and the Miata can get you from Boston to Washington with zip and style in ten hours. The difference is only in the comfort or the pomp, is it not? You might say the same about health care: one plan is more comfortable, more pompous, and more expensive than another, but the end product is the same.

There are, to be sure, minor differences. One HMO may offer more coverage of routine items—vaccinations, common prescription drugs, care for minor illnesses—and another cover catastrophic illness better. One is more convenient. Another uses a prestigious hospital. But don't you still get penicillin if you get a strep throat? Lay out the prospectus honestly. Let the market decide. Medical care is a legitimate consumer choice.

Or is it?

To me, health care is different. First, it concerns a universal need. You can live without a car or with a cheap one—it is your choice—but chances are your life will require you at some time to have medical care. It may not be your choice. It might be routine maintenance—vaccinations, clearance to work, approval for life insurance. It might be more. You might be hit by the speeding sports car. You never know.

Second, with a purchase, you can plan for when you make it, decide how much you wish to pay, inform yourself about the product's qualities, and walk away from the salesperson if you don't like what you hear. But if you develop chest pain in the middle of the night, you may have to trust someone, perhaps someone you have not yet met, to diagnose your condition and to decide to prescribe a pain reliever or a coronary bypass operation. You cannot easily acquire the knowledge that will allow you independently to select what is best. The circumstances are such that you have to delegate to your doctor the responsibility either to dismiss your complaint as trivial or to regard it as life-threatening, to spend a few pennies or several thousand dollars (of the insurance pool's money) on your behalf. If you are in your hometown, if you can speak and think, and if you have the time, you have some flexibility in selecting your doctor or health plan, but most people cannot make an independent judgment about cost-effectiveness, especially in the middle of the night. If you are insured, you don't worry too much about the cost anyway, because you will not directly pay the bill.

Third, unlike many consumer decisions, medical choices will be for a long time. You should hope for this. You want your doctor to know your medical history; you want to trust him; you share your most intimate secrets with your doctor; and you want him to use this accumulated information if you should once again develop late-night chest pain five years from now, and you want him to be available and you want continuity of care.

This is one of the worst parts about having cost as a criterion in selecting a health plan. Your employer may pick a different, more cost-effective plan next year, forcing you to go to a new set of doctors. Or you might change jobs and in that way have to change plans. Your doctor may be fired from your HMO because his treatment decisions cost too much or because he told you more than the HMO wants you to hear.* The HMO may change its rules, may consolidate with another company, or may go out of business. This is not fantasy. All these things have recently happened. Continuity is not guaranteed in managed care.

A fourth reason health care differs from other consumer purchases is that it is the only purchase of services we make that might immediately fail and nonetheless be top-rated. A new car has a warranty, and you can get your money back if a piston cracks before you have driven 50,000 miles. By contrast, medical care is successful when it prevents death and when it cures disease, but it comes without warranty. Not all of your

---

*See S. Woolhandler and D. U. Himmelstein, "Extreme Risk—The New Corporate Proposition for Physicians," *New England Journal of Medicine*, 1995, 333: 1706–7.

body parts can be replaced or saved from harm. There are incurable diseases. Sooner or later everyone will die. It is not often obvious whether failure in treatment comes because the doctor lacks—or is prohibited from applying—necessary skills or because, in that year, in that place, it is that person's time to die. I can give you long explanations, replete with Latin and Greek words, and much technical detail, but I don't really know why Nick d'Abruzzi died at twenty-eight, another patient at forty-three, and a third at ninety, all of the same disease. Why did one patient die suddenly at home the evening of the day we completed the most detailed cardiac studies we knew how to do, all of which showed her to be normal? The technical answers to these questions describe the patient, but they do not explain. To describe how someone dies is not to tell you why.

We have good and universal criteria by which to judge whether a car purchase is good. The car works well or it does not. It is big enough or it is not. Comfortable enough or not. The amount we paid for it is reasonable or not. We know people who have made similar purchases. We can compare our experiences with theirs. The criteria for defining a good medical purchase are less clear. A patient who dies may have received the best medical treatment available. Consider one man, thirty-three years old, who on day one started coughing. He saw our best chest physician on day three, was in the hospital receiving intravenous antibiotics that very night. What appeared to all the doctors to be pneumonia did not respond to treatment. He had a lung biopsy, and a new diagnosis, by day seven: Wegener's granulomatosis, rare, potentially lethal, treatable with medicine, which we started that night. Despite the intensive-care unit and every bit of technology we had, he died on day ten. To us, it was unheard of to lose a patient so quickly from this disease. We reviewed the case in depth several times—all the clinical findings and all the autopsy results. We had missed nothing, we had made the correct diagnosis as fast as was humanly possible and begun the curative treatment with no delay, but his disease did not respond. Our conclusion: superb medicine, horrible outcome.

Another patient may receive very poor service and yet value it highly. A lady had been treated by her personal physician for a decade for rheumatoid arthritis until gout deposits crushed her spinal cord. Emergency neurosurgery partly saved the day. It was then obvious to us that she had never had rheumatoid arthritis: the entire time it had been gout, a completely treatable disease. Lying paralyzed in bed, she nonetheless believed that she had been well served. In fact, she concluded that her rheumatoid arthritis had miraculously disappeared, and that gouty arthritis had supervened. Horrible medicine, deeply appreciated.

People are less alike than cars. Suppose you wake in the middle of the night with chest pain. You probably know someone who had the same symptoms. Within twenty-four hours your friend underwent a coronary bypass operation and was apparently cured. You tell this to your doctor, but he dismisses your advice. You probably don't know that your friend had a single blockage in the main coronary artery, while you have many diffusely narrowed arteries deep within the heart muscle. You do not know that your friend's problem could be treated by surgery but that yours cannot. You may be unhappy with your doctor. You may not understand that you and your friend do not have the same disease. To you this is a Miata versus SL 600 decision. To your doctor it is automobile versus living-room carpet. Who is the best judge of the worth of your medical purchase? Can you really choose? Can your employer, or your HMO?

It is a little easier if you make your choices methodically, when you are not under stress, when you can ask questions and seek other opinions. It is not easier if there is no clear agreement about what to do. Are you considering a hip-replacement operation? Criteria to decide when this should be done are not very clear. One doctor may give highest priority to your pain, another to your walking ability, a third to your age and your other health problems. A friend of mine, a professor in her early fifties, on her feet all day, decided that pain relief and the ability to stand up to lecture were important to her. She and her orthopedist agreed to replace her hip. Her health plan said no, because she was too young. She did not meet the health plan's criteria for surgery. Whose opinion should prevail? (She and her doctor successfully contested the health plan's ruling. Her opinion held sway.)

If the answer is to proceed with the surgery, the second part of the question, how you select types of replacement—between Miata and the SL 600, as it were—is more complex. One hip surgeon may recommend a cemented ("glued"-in) hip replacement, another an uncemented ("bony ingrowth") one, and a third the replacement of only the thighbone but not the pelvic part of the hip. Chances are that the different recommendations reflect the surgeons' personal styles, not that the specific procedure is best for *you*. Chances are that you do not have the specialized knowledge to know which option is both good and cost-effective. Unlike with the Miata–SL 600 decision, you have little information to help you choose. Your aesthetic sense is a poor guide. Eventually you choose because you like one surgeon or one hospital better than another. This is a consumer choice, of course, but, unless you are unusually thorough, it is not one based on important elements of the services offered.

Cost-effectiveness—assigning value for service—is a time-honored rating system. It works best if you have a clear definition of "value" and, for that matter, of "service." Value-for-service judgments do not work well in individual medical-care encounters, and they work much better if you measure the value that a service has had to many people over a long enough time to identify bad outcomes. *Consumer Reports* will probably tell you what percentage of Miatas are still on the road after ten years, but in medicine we have few data that tell us unambiguously what works best, at lowest cost, *for a long time*. In fact, cost-effectiveness measurement is a very new medical science.

To measure value there must be an agreed definition of the term. Economists equate value with money. They measure medical value by the percentage of people returned to the workforce, or by reduced future medication costs. Consider Joe, who slips on the ice and breaks his ankle; he loses five days of work then and a few more days when he visits the doctor to be checked and to have his cast removed. There may be an ambulance fee, a few X-rays, and some doctors' fees. The taxes he pays, and the money he spends in the community when he is back at work, more than pay for the cost of his treatment. The treatment is cost-effective.

Now compare Joe with Hattie, a woman in her late eighties, homebound, cared for by her sisters but able to go to the kitchen and the bathroom on her own. She slips on a loose rug and breaks her hip. If she stays in bed, it will heal, in months. If she has surgery, she will be able to walk in one or two days. Unoperated on, she will be in considerable pain. It will not be expensive to keep her at home—she is there any-way—and in bed. No need to hire nurses: let her sisters tend to her feeding and toileting needs. From an economic point of view there is no need to repair the hip. At her age, she may not live long anyway. To repair her hip will cost an ambulance, a hospitalization, an operation, many X-rays, and physical therapy. Not much value for the dollar here. Unless you count value by her reduced pain, by her ability to get to the bathroom unaided. Hattie does. Her sisters do. But Hattie's needs, as opposed to Joe's, are often ignored in cost-effectiveness debates.

One of the ways to get around this confusion is to perform an exercise called utility analysis. Utility analysis is a new way of looking at values. Its techniques enable us, it is said, to translate abstract concepts like pain into dollars. That translation might generously be called imperfect, but it is a start. In a utility-analysis study, patients, many of whom are suffering from the same, easily defined complaint—pain, for instance, or walking disability—are given a standard gamble: "How much," they are asked, "would you pay to be pain-free? Or to walk again?" Or perhaps the gamble is calculated in years of life instead of dollars. "How many years shorter a life would you accept to be without pain?" One person might put her highest value on living long enough to see a child married; another might choose to have no pain. Numerical values are assigned to each choice—how much to walk, to go to the toilet alone, to leave the house, to entertain friends, to participate in sports, to read—and the answers are factored into a value-for-service equation. When the questions are asked, the answers are sometimes surprising.

No doctor should ever presume what a patient will choose. I, personally, would not like to have my fingers amputated and I think most people agree with me. I have seen patients facing amputations plead, heartbreakingly, to wait just one more day; maybe the finger can still be saved. But one day, I vividly recall, I had put on a grim face to tell a very meticulous elderly woman that we wanted to amputate her index finger. "So what," she replied, with no evident concern. "I have plenty more." Her value for that finger was approximately zero dollars. Mine would have been more.

Now what about the definition of the word "service"? There is the department-store aspect of service, easy to measure: waiting time, pleasantness of the encounter, satisfaction with the apparent outcome. But pleasant service is not the same as good medical care. Granted, marked deviations from an expected outcome will eventually be seen. A badly missed diagnosis, like an unsuspected cancer, like gout deposits crushing the spinal cord, will in time be obvious. Gross medical incompetence will stand out, but not much less.

Without signposts, it is hard to distinguish between superb and pedestrian care. What if your doctor does not know that a new (but expensive) antibiotic is more effective for stomach ulcers than the cheaper antacids he recommends? You will get better with both treatments. Your risk of recurrence, of a later complication, perhaps a very expensive one, will be much higher with the cheap prescription, but this will not be apparent to you at the time. Which prescription is most cost-effective? I would say the expensive one, since it offers a permanent cure. Your HMO has an annual budget to report. It might choose the other. It is cheap, and you feel well on the day you fill out your satisfaction questionnaire.

What if your general doctor mistakenly treats your arthritis with cortisone and the health-plan thinks that specialist consultation for such a "simple" problem is too costly? Your joint pains will disappear. Cortisone's side effects will not show up for years. If a bone fractures, or if you develop cataracts, you may not even realize that these complications are the result of your prior treatment. By my reckoning, you will have been badly served, but you may not think so if the doctor and staff were pleasant and efficient at the time. Nor may your health plan or your employer, because they have saved money in the short term.* Besides, says the HMO, some other HMO may have to pay for the complications five or ten years from now. Cost-effectiveness is measured at the end of the fiscal year, not at the end of a life.

Who decides whether a doctor's service is good or bad anyway, and by what criteria? You? The HMO? Your employer, who hires the HMO? The answers to these questions are not self-evident. Check your policy. Check with your employer. It may be any of the above. It may be none. I think it should be you.

Consumer rules do not work for medical care. Its special circumstances, its universality of need, the emergent nature of many of its decisions, the technical knowledge needed to make decisions, the abstract values you personally hold, the long-term outcomes, and the inevitability of eventual failure all mean that we need more than consumer rules, more than cost-effectiveness measures, to restructure our delivery of health care.

We have to agree about our priorities. We have to select what we want for the individual and for the population as a whole. We have to choose priorities that are both abstract and concrete. We have to identify those that are moral and right. Then we must protect them when fiscal tools, like value for service, take center stage.

*Employers appear to pay little attention to quality measures and great attention to cost when selecting an HMO, according to David Segal in *The Washington Post*, January 19, 1996. But others think that employers are beginning to look at quality. See Stuart Auerbach, *The Washington Post*, March 1, 1996, and Maggie Mahar, *Barron's*, March 4, 1996.

THE COST OF AGE

Consider this abstract question: Is it right to spend 30 percent of Medicare dollars on Americans' last year of life? Put differently, is it right that people over the age of sixty-five, according to the Census Bureau, account for more than one of every four of our nation's health-care dollars?

Rethink the question in a personal way: Your eighty-five-year-old mother (or even you yourself) is well and self-sufficient. Your family ties are close. Your mother is enthusiastic about seeing her first great-grandchild (your grandchild), whose birth is expected several months from now. Tonight she calls you and says that her chest hurts and she cannot breathe.

How do you respond? Do you say, "Mom, at your age, I don't want to waste any money"? Or do you say, "Let's call your doctor"?

You make the second choice. The doctor thinks it is a heart attack and admits your mother to the nearest hospital. This costs about nine hundred dollars per day, again according to the Census Bureau. She has an irregular heartbeat; the doctors recommend that she go to the coronary-care unit (two thousand dollars per day). Medicare covers most of the expense. The next day she feels better and is eager to go home. The doctors, however, tell you that her heart rate changed and they inserted a temporary pacemaker through her vein. Her heart works well with the pacemaker, but if the doctors remove it, she will immediately become bed-bound and breathless, and she will frequently faint; she probably will not die. They tell you further that they want to put in a permanent pacemaker. With it, she can return to normal health, except that she will need to visit both her regular doctor and a cardiologist frequently.

This high-technology pacemaker costs more than a thousand dollars. It requires a surgical procedure—another few thousand dollars added to the hospital bill. The follow-up monitoring will be expensive, too. Your mother told the doctors that she would like to know that you agree to the surgery, so they ask for your consent. (This scenario is very common.)

There are several questions. The first is: When you have to make hard decisions—spending money for care of the elderly is one—will you make the same choice for those close to you as you do when you think abstractly of elderly people as a group? Is saying no to high technology for octogenarians the same as saying no to your mother? A second question: If your mother, sound of mind, says she wants the pacemaker, do you have the right to say no? Does her doctor? (I am not talking here of a technology with only equivocal benefit, or of somebody with a hopeless prognosis.) How about legislative or rule-making bodies? Can they say no? If the state told you that there was a limit on spending for persons over eighty and that the limit meant no pacemaker, would you accept? Japan spends half of what the United States does on medical care, and it does so by rationing services to octogenarians. Japan's choice makes a difference: almost 20 percent more eighty-year-old Americans than Japanese live five more years. What Americans spend on health care for the elderly does buy them longer life.*

What if no publicly accountable body, and not you, and not even your mother, but a for-profit business, with anonymous

*See N. Ikegami and J. C. Campbell, "Medical Care in Japan," *New England Journal of Medicine*, 1995, 333:1295–99; and K. G. Manton and J. W. Vaupel, "Survival After the Age of 80 in the United States, Sweden, France, England, and Japan," *New England Journal of Medicine*, 1995, 333: 1232–35.

decision makers, decides to say no to your mother? The choice not to treat her might be made by an insurance company, health maintenance organization, or maybe her employer. Not by her, not by you, not by her doctor. These organizations, after all, set the limits of medical care. Under the fee-for-service idea, personal choice is possible. Indeed, Medicare might permit your mother, at eighty-five, to make a choice that might be forbidden to you at half her age. Does her personal choice have a higher value than does cost of her care? Is personal choice without limits? One answer to this conundrum is that choice cannot be delegated. Elderly patients must decide for themselves.

Old age and chronic illness are the reasons the American health-care bill is so high. It costs more to care for the old than for the young. With each decade of life, the health-care bill grows. The chart from the Census Bureau on the next page shows the annual per capita cost of health care in the United States at each adult decade. A person twenty to twenty-nine years old costs only about $350 per year; a person eighty and above costs eight times more.

At any period of time, those who are employed, healthy, and young, pay most of the bill with their taxes and insurance premiums. We have chosen to pay for medical care this way. It is the purpose of Medicare, Medicaid, and Social Security. We pay taxes so that the government will provide all of us with a safety net. The point of all insurance—theft and fire and collision as well as health insurance—is that many subscribers share the cost, knowing that by bad luck each one may someday be in need. It is part of our social contract. It is the very reason why we insure.

Except: it is an individual choice to insure property for a lot or a little. It is not individual choice to have an illness that is low-cost or one that is dear.

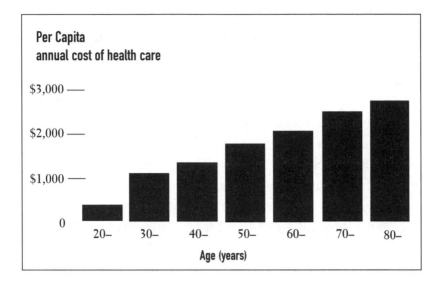

Except: you probably will not crash your car. It is unlikely that your house will burn down. But it is very likely that you will one day need medical care.

The cost per person for insurance is calculated according to a simple formula:

$$\text{Cost per person (premium)} = \left(\text{Cost per claim} \times \frac{\text{Number of claimants}}{\text{Number of contributors}}\right) + \text{Profit}$$

In other words, the cost of the premium goes up if the cost for each claim, the number of claimants, or the profit rises, or if the total number of contributors goes down.

The cost of health-insurance premiums is increasing. Why? The reason is not the cost per claim nor is it the profit. The reason is that the ratio of claimants to contributors is changing. The ratio is increasing. We are not in a steady state. With each passing day we have more claimants and fewer contributors, because we now have smaller families and live much longer. In 1970 there were 5.3 people between twenty and sixty-five years of age for each person over sixty-five; by 2020 there will be only 3.7. If the annual cost per person does not change, between 1970 and 2020 we will need a 46 percent increase in each contributor's bill *just to stay even*, as the Census Bureau table on the next page makes clear. Of course, at some point the ratio of elderly to young will again become stable. When we reach a steady state again, costs will no longer rise.

Another set of figures makes the reason for the high cost of medicine very clear. The proportion of America that is sixty-five or more years old was barely 10 percent in 1970; by 2025 that proportion will have doubled, and the proportion eighty-five and older will have trebled. Consider that in 1970 the average age at death was seventy-one; in 2010 it will be seventy-eight. The Medicare population today uses 35 percent of our federal health-care dollars. But a projection based purely on demographic changes shows that those over sixty-five will use nearly twice that amount in 2025 than they did in 1970; the only difference is the proportion of the population that is old. Where people once died in their sixties, they now live until their eighties and nineties, with chronic illnesses. That we support the chronically ill, the elderly, our parents, is a glorious declaration of the type of humane and civil people we are. That we do not acknowledge that we have *chosen* to do this, and that this choice is costly, is the problem.

The Japanese answer to the problem, as we have seen, is to ration care for the elderly. The elderly, the argument goes, have lived their lives; they should now withdraw and leave the nation's resources to their heirs. To accept this solution you must believe that sixty-five-year-olds should be forbidden their prostatectomies, breast biopsies, cataract surgeries, blood-pressure medicines, hip replacements, heart and bone and joint medicines, and the rest. How otherwise could you ration their care?

I see a movie called *Logan's Run* from time to time in reruns

Year	Number of Consumers (aged 65+) for every 10 contributors (20–65)	$ Annual cost per consumer	$ Annual cost per contributor
1970	53	2000	377
1980	50	2000	399
1990	47	2000	428
2020	37*	2000	550

*18–65, not 20–65.

on television. In the movie everyone reaching the age of thirty is invited to move, in a process called "renewal," to a higher level of life. The invitees go eagerly—to be killed, it turns out—being unaware that death is what "renewal" means. Logan is a policeman whose job is to catch those who do not want to go. He discovers the secret of "renewal" and himself runs away. The argument that the elderly should surrender their rights to health care is like that of *Logan's Run*. You are old. It is time for you to die.

I pray that we have not yet reached that point. For one thing, even if a don't-treat-the-elderly argument could be made and agreed on, the other, major point I am trying to make would be lost. It is not just the old who cost money. It is also those preparing to become old. In the table above I called people over age sixty-five "consumers" of medical care and those under sixty-five "contributors." This convenient dichotomy simplified my calculations, but the terms "consumer" and "contributor" are not correct. Young people also use large amounts of health care, and not all the old are consumers of it.

People buy medical services for most of their lives. We buy health care in our twenties for our families—think of obstetrical and pediatric costs. Any group of twenty-year-olds con-

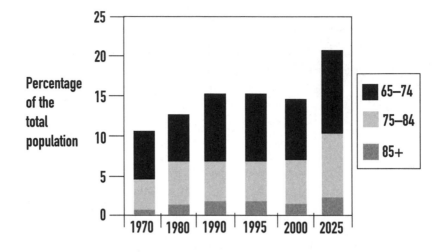

tains a small number of chronically ill people whose individual medical expenses are high and who raise the overall average. In our thirties and forties we invest in medical care to prevent disability. Some in this age group now get blood-pressure treatment, Pap smears, mammograms, prostate tests, and psychiatric evaluations, forestalling more expensive care further on. Forty-year-olds have a larger proportion of people who are chronically ill—diabetics, asthmatics, and others. Among people in their fifties, more of the same and a still larger proportion now chronically ill: a measurable number of people with cancer, coronaries, strokes, arthritis, alcoholism, emphysema, schizophrenia and other costly diseases. Disability among people in their fifties is very common. Indeed, the Census Bureau tells us that almost *one-quarter* of persons fifty-five to sixty-four years old—still counted in anyone's definition of young—are disabled and receive disability assistance. These people are not, for the most part, homebound. They are people you know—many of them—who use canes, former football players with bad knees, people with back pain, chest disease, visual and hearing loss, mental illness, drug dependence, and lesser ills.

Chronic, not acute, illness among both the young *and* the old is the major reason we seek medical care. Most of the money we spend alleviates noncritical chronic disabilities that last a long time for both young and old.

The average cost *per illness* is less, not more, than it once was. In the 1940s my grandfather spent six weeks in the hospital when he had his coronary attack; today he might spend three days. But the average cost *per person* is higher because over a long life span people use many more services than they ever did. My grandfather died in his sixties. Today he would live into his eighties. In those extra twenty years he probably would have a bypass operation, a prostatectomy, a cataract operation, and a hip replacement. In the 1940s my grandfather paid his own way; if he had not, he would have received little care. Today everybody receives care. More people, more claims, more claims per person—old age and chronic illness are the major reasons our health-care bill is so high. But who among us would now challenge long survival? Who would now turn back the clock?

There is no single point, no single age, at which costs per person suddenly rise. As the chart on page 217 shows, *three-quarters* of what we spend today we spend for people *under the age of sixty-five*. The young are not only "contributors" but "consumers," too. Although we worry about a future when the cost for medical care for the old will approach half the total bill, we are anxious about the cost of health care *today*. If there were no Medicare at all—*nothing* for persons over sixty-five— federal taxes would be low; *but the doctor bills for the young will not change*, and the cost to employers will not decrease. In fact, if workers were unable to rely on Medicare, they might demand more protection from their pensions, and the cost to employers might go up.

In thinking about rationing health care for the elderly,

should we choose an arbitrary age, say eighty? Octogenarians are only marginally more expensive than are septuagenarians, who themselves are little different from sexagenarians. Octogenarians account for only 12 percent of the total national bill. To pick an age at which we would prohibit spending, we would have to draw a very arbitrary, very unfair line, a sort of Do Not Resuscitate order for elderly *well* people. *Logan's Run*, one notch higher.

What would we revoke from the elderly? "Big ticket" items—heart transplants, dialysis—is a common response. But these account for only a small fraction of medicine's total cost. Eliminating the "big ticket" items might save money, true: new high-technology treatments for heart attacks make the cost of treating them rise four percentage points above the inflation rate each year; if you assign a dollar value to the added life, though, the new treatments reduce the cost 1 percent per year—an eye-of-the-beholder argument if there ever was one. Most of the medical expense for elderly patients goes to the amelioration of nonlethal disabilities, "little ticket" items. Yet these, too, are costly in a less dramatic way. Nursing care is labor-intensive and not cheap.

So the cost to care for our elderly citizens is high because there are many of them, not because there is individual great expense or because vast amounts of high technology are used.* In fact, *on a per person basis*, the elderly are cheaper to care for now than in the past. Because disability has declined, Med-

---

*See E. J. and L. L. Emanuel, "The Economics of Dying: The Illusion of Costs Savings at the End of Life," *New England Journal of Medicine*, 1994, 330:540–44; J. Lubitz, J. Beebe, and C. Baker, "Longevity and Medicare Expenditures," *New England Journal of Medicine*, 1995, 332:999–1003, and A. M. Kramer, "Health Care for Elderly Persons—Myths and Realities," *New England Journal of Medicine*, 1995, 1027–29.

icare saved $200 billion between 1982 and 1995, as Gina Ko-
lata reported in *The New York Times* in 1996. If we were to
withdraw "big ticket" care from the elderly, we would not
achieve important savings. Nor will we ever, unless we ask people with poor sight, or poor mobility, or poor hearing, or weak
hearts or lungs to fend for themselves. Unless we take away
their canes and hearing aids and eyeglasses and condemn them
to suffer for the (many) last years of their lives.

Another argument has it that much expense is wasted on
unwanted, futile terminal care. Let the elderly die in peace,
the argument goes, let them die a little earlier, with dignity—
and much less cost.

But again, the doctors' choices and the available modern
technology that prolongs (meaningless) life are not important
cost items. Without doctors, old people do not die rapidly.
Old age is not a sustained lethal disease that medical intervention keeps at bay. Old age is more like (apologies to Ste-
phen Jay Gould) punctuated equilibrium. It is stable chronic
illness, or disability, interrupted by bouts of acute, most often
nonlethal illness: a mild heart attack, a small stroke, a fractured
hip. These events take their toll but do not inevitably kill.
With routine, low-technology care, most of the elderly survive
such bouts, and they do not spend long periods dying in
intensive-care wards.

Suppose that, to save money, we did not treat elderly patients during these acute bouts of illness. We have to realize
that surviving, untreated, they would generate costs in other
ways. Without a walker, or without a home health assistant, a
disabled person might need expensive nursing-home care. The
logic holds for high-cost items as well. A hip replacement costs
$10,000. In rationed care, with hip replacement forbidden to
those over eighty, an octogenarian unable to walk might spend
$20,000 *each year* in a nursing home. So withdrawing care from

the elderly will not save money. On the contrary, because of additional social costs, it may cost the nation more.

Imagine that a (health insurance) business contracts to provide services for ten thousand subscribers for a fixed fee. Imagine that only a small number of the subscribers actually use the services. Imagine that the business spends one thousand dollars to provide those services each year and your aim is to reduce this by half. What you do not know is how that thousand dollars was spent—as ten cents for each one of the subscribers, or one dollar each for a thousand, or five hundred dollars apiece for only two people. You need to know the number of users before you can compute the average cost and determine how best to save.

The analogy explains why our health-care debate is so bewildering. In popular fantasy, our Medicare and health-care costs are five-hundred-dollar items for two of the ten thousand users. This concept is very rousing in public debate. It lends itself to an easy solution. Cut one of the two items: 9,999 people will be pleased and only one will lose out.

In truth, the number of users is far more than two. There are very few—maybe even no—five-hundred-dollar items. There may be some dollar items, maybe even a five-dollar item, but most health-care charges are equivalent to a penny, a nickel, a dime, a quarter spent on a thousand, five thousand, or all ten thousand subscribers. The payments are dribbled out as small items for home assistance, nursing homes, medications, more frequent doctor visits and short-term hospitalizations. Cut the bill in half and you deprive many people, not just a few. There will be five thousand people pleased that you achieved the savings and five thousand dismayed—maybe even one thousand pleased and nine thousand dismayed.

To achieve any substantial savings at all in our nation's medical expenses, we will have to ration for the young as well as the old. The choice will be the same: to restrict access to high-technology items used by few patients, or to low-technology items used by many. Only the latter will save much money. What must be rationed, and how it should be rationed, must be consciously chosen.

I do not accept the idea that rationing must be only for those who are old. I do not accept it for a moral reason: it is wrong to exclude classes of people. And I do not accept the idea for a practical reason: it will not save enough.

7

THE FUTURE

COST SAVING

Here is a schoolbook exercise. Your task is to reduce the medical-care budget, all of it if possible, or at least the federal part. Most of the data you need to know are in the table on pages 227 and 228. The total cost of medical care in the United States in 1993, to take a recent year, was almost a trillion dollars. Use these numbers. See what you can do. There are no rules. You are on your own. I suggest that you try to save a large amount, say 20 percent or more. Keep in mind that the costs will worsen in the future, as the proportion of the aged in our society grows. Big cuts now will be better than small.

On second thought, there is one rule: when you cut an item, do not cut it just because the number is big or because you think from the item's name that the money is poorly spent. Think about what that dollar now buys. Itemize what you will have to take away. Consider what alternatives remain.

Item	Percentage of total health-care costs	Percent of federal health-care budget
Government total	44	100
Hospital care	35	
Physicians' services	20	
Medicare total	19	40
Age >65	12	28
Hospitals, general	9	20
Disabled	2	4
Outpatient clinic	1	3
Home health care	<1	<1
Medicaid total	14	32
Disabled	4	10
Age >65	4	8
AFDC	3	8
Hospitals, general	3	7
Nursing homes	3	7
Pharmaceuticals	1	2
Mental retardation	1	2
Home health care	1	1
Hospitals, mental	<1	1
Pharmaceuticals and devices	8	
Unintentional injury	8	
Nursing home	8	
Administration	5	
Mental health	3	
Home care	3	
Workman's compensation	2	5
Veterans, medical care	2	4
Research (public)	1	3
Vision	1	
Substance abuse, medical	1	

Item	Percentage of total health-care costs	Percent of federal health-care budget
Firearms, medical	1	
Alcohol, medical	<1	

The first column lists the items. The second column shows the percentage of the total national cost for each, and the third column, where relevant, the percentage of the cost to the federal government. (The table is not inclusive. Some of the numbers are estimates, and there is overlap. The figures for alcohol and substance abuse, for instance, may include patients with both conditions. Administration does not include administrative costs in a doctor's bill: the doctors' office administrative costs, malpractice insurance, etc.)

The table shows percentages. It could have shown dollars, but then the larger picture disappears. The medical cost of alcoholism is $8 billion a year, which sounds like an immense sum, but it is less than 1 percent of the total bill. Or how about medical research? Also 1 percent. These items are nickels and dimes—or, to be more literal, pennies—of the health-care dollar. Better to stick with percentages, so you know each item's relative place.

Now do the assignment. Your task is to find the items to cut that will allow the best health care for everyone, that will be politically feasible, and that will be moral as well. You should make your own choices for each item: to reduce its cost or reduce its use.

A good place to start might be the most expensive items: hospital care, physicians' services, Medicare, and Medicaid. A good strategy might be to hunt for and abolish waste. HMO executives and many politicians (though few doctors) believe that there is still a lot of fat to trim. I myself think this is unlikely. Have you been in a hospital lately? Did you see signs of excess? If so, why are patients discharged too rapidly? Why are there too few nurses? Why is the equipment shoddy and the buildings in disrepair?

No matter. Assume that resources are indeed squandered. Assume that better management will be able to save 10 percent of the bill. Cuts like this may eliminate redundancy, but they will mean more hospitals closing, even shorter hospital stays for patients, fewer tests, no intensive-care units or hospital admissions for some patients, and more hospital personnel dismissed. Hospitals will find it cheaper to hire their own physicians rather than permitting your personal doctor to authorize admissions to their beds. Physicians employed by the hospitals will forbid expensive tests. They will discharge patients at the hospital administrator's command.* Perhaps physicians' assistants will do most of the doctors' work. Perhaps aides, not nurses, will staff the floors. If this is satisfactory, go ahead. Cut hospital costs by 10 percent. You will save about 3 percent of the total health-care bill. That is an important but not a huge amount. A good start.

Another option might be to reduce the cost of physicians' services, which represents 20 percent of the bill. You can do this by cutting the number of services doctors dispense. Your pneumonia is not improving fast enough? Your doctor wants another chest X-ray to see why? Not allowed. The rules allow only two X-rays per case. Alternatively, you can have patients pay less for each service. Some physicians might work for lower pay. Or deny patients the "privilege" of specialist care, since specialists cost more than nonspecialists. Having generalists provide all of our medical care might save money, so long as we are willing to accept the lesser skill and tolerate possible

*See R. M. Wachter and L. Goldman, "The Emerging Role of 'Hospitalists' in the American Health Care System," *New England Journal of Medicine*, 1996, 335:514–17.

errors by those whose training is broad but not deep. How much will all this save? Do the arithmetic. If you cut physicians' services by a Draconian one-third, the savings will amount to 6 percent of the nation's total medical bill.

I do not argue that doctors are now paid appropriately. I am very much aware that their fees, not to say their outright greed, escalated in the 1980s, when many of them set the highest possible "usual and customary" fee. You can say that doctors deserve to have their fees brought down. An argument for lowering the level of doctors' income has merit. Still, overall, their incomes are not so outrageous, and the average doctor works 52 hours per week, the rest of the working nation 35. The mean net income for all of them is $182,400 (for family-practice doctors, $121,200).

However, physicians' income represents only about half the cost of their services. What about their office assistants, their landlords, and their malpractice insurers—which together claim the other half? They will not happily share a one-third cut. The proposed savings will have to come entirely from physicians' personal incomes.

Cutting physicians' services by a whopping 33 percent would cut the average doctor's net pretax income by two-thirds and lower a family practitioner's by 50 percent.* In many cases this would reduce them to poverty levels. Physicians will surely accept some loss of income, but not a decrease of this amount. To be reasonable, cuts will have to be much smaller, but then of course savings are that much less.

I know that an argument to maintain doctors' incomes will gain no sympathy—I have had too many fingers poked into my

---

*I calculated these figures by adding doctors' net income and professional expenses (which are, as a mean, $183,100 ($190,500 for family doctors), taking one-third of the total and subtracting it from net income.

chest to imagine otherwise. But we cannot be sure that physicians will continue to work their long hours, that students will apply to medical school, that there will be no doctor strikes, or that the nation's preeminence in medicine will continue if we so drastically reduce doctors' pay. It would be an experiment, pure and simple, the results of which are unknown.

Another way to save would be to reduce administrative costs. Because we have many insurers, each with many confusing rules, because all sorts of treatments require prior approval of the insurance companies and each patient encounter is a separate transaction, the system generates huge administrative bills. Private doctors have added another person to their offices just to handle the paperwork. The cost of having so many insurers is twenty-five cents on every health-care dollar. A single-payer system would surely save money: $118 billion per year, 15 percent of our total bill.*

Canada has cheaper health care than we do, though it is rising, and a single-payer system. (It also has fewer guns, less violence, less poverty, and no uninsured people.) An American patient costs twice as much as a Canadian one does. Canada has mostly primary-care doctors; we have many specialists. Canada uses less medical technology than we do. Can we emulate Canada and reduce our cost? Recently a team of Canadian and American doctors compared health costs in the two nations. They studied a single chronic illness, lupus. As I have tried to show in this book, the prudent treatment of lupus

---

*See S. Woolhandler and D. U. Himmelstein, "The Deteriorating Administrative Efficiency in the U.S. Health Care System," *New England Journal of Medicine*, 1991, 324:1253–58; See also I. Hellander, D. U. Himmelstein, S. Woolhandler, and S. Wolfe, "Health Care Paper Chase, 1993: The Cost to the Nation, the States, and the District of Columbia," *International Journal of Health Services*, 1994, 24:1–9.

requires cleverness in the use of resources over time. They looked at each cost item, every test, every prescription, every office visit, and every hospitalization. They found that costs were different not because American doctors overused technology or specialty care, but because American doctors charged more for every test and because the American population is so diverse. Nonwhite patients (more numerous in the United States) have poorer prognoses and higher costs.*

Compared with Americans, Canadians use more, not fewer, medical services. They make more emergency-room visits, probably because of delayed or superficial care of problems not well resolved in the hospital or office. They take more medication. Their hospital stays are twice as long as ours. Specialist care, a supposed reason for America's high costs, makes no difference at all.

If American doctors' charges had been as low as the Canadians', the cost for American patients would have been much *less* than those in Canada. (Still, one should not get too comfortable with the idea that, since Canadian doctors accept lower fees, American doctors will as well. Canadian doctors have recently gone on strike.) American medical care, the authors concluded, is *more* efficient than Canada's. Its costs, they said, reflect our demography and the prices we pay, not the use of specialists or the manner in which we deliver medical care.

---

*Most of the costs in this category went to care for patients whose kidneys had failed and who needed dialysis. The authors of the study excluded other possible explanations for this result: that the Canadian patients had been better treated, hence less frequently progressed to kidney failure; that they had been worse treated and therefore died when they developed kidney failure. In the United States and Canada (and elsewhere), black patients develop kidney failure more frequently than do whites. Of the American patients 34.5 percent were nonwhite, compared with 16.5 percent of the Canadians.

We do have high costs. The reasons are: we are getting older, we are diverse, we have high professional fees, and we subsidize the rich with Medicare and the middle class with Medicaid. We can reduce waste, we can force fees down, and we can convert to a single-payer system. These will be one-time savings. To enact these reforms will drop the fiscal thermostat a few notches and gain important time. Then the costs will begin escalating again, because the real reason for our rising health-care cost is our changing demography. We are getting older. That change is preordained.

RESTRICTING ACCESS

Perhaps we can find some unnoticed, large, noncritical segment of the current budget, eliminate it, and not have to go through this exercise at all. Reduce our use of high technology, for instance. If we do, will we save very much? Enough to shrink the total health-care bill? We could arbitrarily reduce access to the high-cost miracles: CAT and MRI and PET scans, heart, bone-marrow and liver transplants, gene therapy, and all the technologies that make national news. We can stop trying to save the unsalvageable, the very small premature babies and the "terminally" ill. Administratively it is easy to make these changes. But cutting back on high technology will save little. High-technology items are only a small fraction of the total health-care bill. And morally, it is not easy to deny the possibilities that we can now achieve with technology, when there is wide public knowledge of its power. That particular genie will not easily go back in the bottle.

Hospital care is 35 percent of the bill, so should we keep people out of hospitals? Identify hospital services that could be provided at home? Do not assume that these services will not be needed or, at home, will be free. We *can* substitute home health services, but that will still cost money. If we offer no public payment for home services, we leave the ill vulnerable, dependent on the luck of their wealth or poverty. We have done that before. Before 1966, before Medicare. It was not better then.

We could ask everyone to pay more out of pocket, ask for a large "first dollar" payment. If you dent a fender on your car and your collision insurance is $1,000 deductible, you decide whether to do the repair. Could you do the same with your health? Considering the cost, you would probably use fewer services. If many people asked for less, this solution would reduce the total health-care cost. If they did not, high first-dollar payment would simply shift the federal cost to the private pocket. Taxes would not seem so bad, but the medical bills would still enrage.

The poor will suffer more if they have to pay first dollar. To ease their burden, we could compute the first dollar on a sliding scale—a high first dollar for the rich, a smaller one for the poor. But this would require a cumbersome bureaucracy, encourage cheating, and penalize wealth. A high first dollar deductible may make old age a dire time. Before Medicare the elderly lived in dread of the cost of catastrophic illness, nursing-home expenses, and the like. They may do so again.

Medical care by general physicians costs less than specialist medical care. Patients ask for new treatments, and they are usually expensive. The HMO response is to restrict access to these special new techniques, to use a gatekeeper to shut the door. Patients, especially those with chronic diseases, may disagree. Yet to reduce cost, the choice is to restrict or to pay.

Your gatekeeper is likely to be your primary-care doctor. Pay attention: he has two functions. The first is to oversee your medical care. The second is to keep his employer's expenses down. Gatekeepers authorize your access to high-cost medical treatment and specialist care. The gatekeeper policy, intended to motivate physicians to consider costs, creates a prototypical conflict of interest. He is penalized—it costs him money, his own personal money, to seek resources for his sick patients, and he is rewarded when he denies those resources to them.

Unlimited referral to specialists is undeniably wasteful, as is unlimited access to all treatments. The intent of the gatekeeper policy is honorable, but to rely on a doctor to take it out of his own pocket in order to guarantee good patient care is unrealistic. A gatekeeper at personal financial risk is the wrong person to make decisions regarding your care.

An alternative might be a voluntary, personal, supplemental medical insurance, an "I disagree with my gatekeeper" policy that allows second opinions or treatments to those who buy it. This may be feasible, but it seems unwise. Sick people might purchase this supplemental insurance more than well people, and the premium would become unaffordable. Policyholders might use the insurance when it is not needed, which would also drive up premiums.

When the patient wants a consultation and the gatekeeper disagrees, the situation calls for an *independent* referee. Not the courts, which are slow and confrontational, and not an appeals board controlled by the HMO. The arbiter must be quick, independent, and authorized to command. Pooled funds from the industry, with each company being tithed, could support an independent board, which could help HMOs to contain unreasonable demand and patients to control their own lives.

This is the quandary: as individuals, we want access to all the treatments and to all the specialists. And so we should. In no other part of our lives do we deliberately choose a provider with lesser skills. In no other part of our lives do we enthusiastically reject what we have learned. To forbid access to the best in medical care is crazy. But we must restrict access or allow the costs to rise. I suppose there might be a compromise—some increased access, some restrictions—but this does not change the argument, only the quantity of assigned pain.

There might even be a fourth solution: no limitations on access to medical treatment, the same amount of care, but lower *all* the rates, negotiate lower fees for all doctors—say by 30 percent, as has been suggested. Some people may find this fourth a good solution, but I do not, and not just because my own ox would be gored. Many hospitals are now near bankruptcy. Morale among physicians is already low. This might completely destroy the medical skills we now have at our command.

Accept less? Pay for more? How do we choose? One way is not to choose, to be passive, to muddle through, to let the flow of history decide in its own untidy way who will be elected to "accept" less. It will be patients who have bad luck. People who are unemployed and people who are uninsured. People who actually need high-cost medical help and people who the for-profit health care corporations decree will not be served. Patients with "preexisting" conditions or bad "risk profiles" will be turned away. They will be the cherries that will *not* be picked this time, but will be left to rot on the ground.

We could, of course, pay more for our medicine, but I doubt that we will vote for this option. We have so many other calls on our public money—education, safety, shelter, food, infrastructure, defense, and so many other things—that it is unrealistic (not impossible) to argue that health care deserves more.

That leaves the other option, accept less. Reduce services. Retrench. Set limits. Downsize. Call it what you will, it means rationing. And thoughtful rationing means that we must confront some fundamental questions head-on.

8

THE BASIC QUESTIONS

I will follow that system or regimen which, according to my ability and judgment, I consider for the benefit of my patients, and abstain from whatever is deleterious and mischievous . . . Into whatever houses I enter, I will go into them for the benefit of the sick . . .

—The Hippocratic Oath

Fifth century b.c.e.

Thou hast endowed man with the wisdom to relieve the suffering of his brother, to recognize his disorders, to extract the healing substances, to discover their powers and to prepare and to apply them to suit every ill. In Thine Eternal Providence Thou hast chosen me to watch over the life and health of Thy creatures . . . Preserve the strength of my body and of my soul that they ever be ready to cheerfully help and support rich and poor, good and bad, enemy as well as friend. In the sufferer let me see only the human being.

—The Prayer of Maimonides

Twelfth century

The health of my patient will be my first consideration . . . I will maintain the utmost respect for human life.

—The Declaration of Geneva

1948, revised 1983

These are facts:

- Americans live longer now than ever before.
- Much (or most) of our medical care is effective. It helps us to prolong life, lessen pain, and improve our well-being.
- The longer we live, the more we spend for medical care.
- Untreated disabilities are costly, but these costs are often not related to those of medical care.
- HMOs boast of illness *prevention*, but their views are short-term. It would be better called illness *delayed*. Patients who are initially kept healthy by preventive care do age and do, later, die. Health maintenance does not forestall their future medical care.

The facts suggest pessimistic answers to the question: Can we reduce health-care costs? A population that ages will use more health services. No amount of tinkering—curtailing specialty referral, denying tests or treatments, reducing hospital days to a point beyond discomfort—will change this truth. As the American population ages, the cost of medicine will continue to rise.

Unless we ask the most fundamental questions about doctors. Unless we ask: What is the goal of medical care?

For millennia Western society has assigned to doctors, and doctors have enthusiastically accepted, a specific role. For twenty-five hundred years, doctors have vowed to act for the benefit of their patients. For nine hundred years physicians have prayed for the ability to relieve suffering, to help and support each patient, and to see in the sufferer *only* the human being. Fifty years ago, doctors reaffirmed: "The health of my patient will be my first consideration." Thirty-plus years ago,

I and my colleagues took the Oath of Hippocrates, read Maimonides, and accepted the Declaration of Geneva.

My training did not teach, nor did my vows proclaim, that I should treat only those persons for whom a cost-benefit is proved. I took no oath to consider my employer's profit ahead of a patient's needs. Quite the contrary, I did then wholeheartedly swear, and I still freely affirm, that my duty is to relieve suffering for *every* ill. I did then and I do now believe that the patient's health is my first concern.

The high cost of health care thus poses an unthinkable question: Is it time to abandon these ancient oaths? If it costs too much to relieve suffering, do we now call Hippocrates out-of-date and Maimonides passé? Should the new first principle of a physician be: I shall attend only those whom I can cheaply cure?

A doctor's answer must be No.

A doctor still plays the ancient role: to ameliorate, to help, to palliate, to alleviate, to allay, and, if possible, to cure. A doctor's duty still is to be an advocate for his patients, not to bar them from the door. Hippocrates would not have imagined, the Geneva Declaration expressly forbade, an alternative role, in which doctors solitarily choose who will or will not gain access to therapy and select some persons to live and others to die.

I am not oblivious to the cost of medicine. I read newspapers. I watch television and listen to National Public Radio. I read scholarly articles by doctors and economists. I agree that health costs are high. More, I accept that it is my duty to be wise in how I spend medical dollars when I do my work. But as one single doctor, standing beside one single bed, I cannot do the calculus that health policymakers now exact. I cannot make a bedside point-of-service decision to withhold care to save a corporate dollar. My obligation is to argue for and to do what best serves my patient's need. I cannot argue on a patient's behalf and at the same time triage that patient for an industry's gain.

If palliation and mitigation have no value, if medicine's *only* goal is to prevent or cure, if fiscal matters cause us to repudiate Hippocrates, then let this happen only after loud and contentious public debate. Let the whole nation—doctors and patients, parents and children, young and old—hear it shouted aloud: we are now renouncing millennia of devotion to a basic creed of Western civilization. Let the public clearly understand the import of this change and vote its assent. If the public so chooses, I will accept (though not understand) its decree. No tradition is inviolate. Other societies value health care less, and so can we. Even great ideas must and will change.

As must words. Without Hippocrates and Maimonides, the name "physician" would lose its meaning. In its place we would have to substitute a more apposite term. When you waken at night with chest pain, do not call a doctor. Call instead your fiscal triage officer. Do not ask him if he can help. Ask him why palliation and mitigation, even kindness, no longer have value. Ask rather: Is there profit in curing me?

Why do people save money? Is it for their children or for themselves? Does an older citizen keep money in the bank to provide for his own food, housing, and health in old age, or does he keep it to provide his children a legacy? A man who retires in 1995 contributed $30,691 to Medicare but he will typically get back $80,442 after adjustment for inflation, *The New York Times* tells us.

Many believe that government has a duty to care for our

old citizens. In anticipation of this help, some middle-class families transfer their savings to their children, giving them an advance legacy, so that they themselves qualify for Medicaid nursing-home care. They argue that they do not want to burden their children with debt—an honorable wish. But is it right *both* to give the children an advance legacy *and* to release them from the burden of paying for their parents' care? There should be a choice: to pay for elder care through taxes (government caring for the old) or through personal savings (less or no inheritance for the children). The alternatives are morally equivalent. The issues are whether both give parity between rich and poor, and who—the patient or the government—is accountable.

With Medicare as with Social Security, rich and poor benefit equally. It might be different. We could ask the rich to pay for their own care. We could means-test medical assistance. We could provide public medical support only for the poor. Then the rich would be paying out of pocket for their own care *and* out of taxes for care of the poor. This is a policy that forces tax-regulated, involuntary charity.

If we chose this policy, the *federal* health bill would be much lower, but the *total* health-care cost would be the same, with great individual disparity even among the rich. One rich old person might die suddenly on a golf course, never having spent a penny for medical care, and his family will inherit all his wealth. Another might develop a lingering illness, spend his fortune on personal care, and leave his family nothing. When the government subsidizes health care for both the rich and the poor, medical happenstance does not determine a family's fiscal fate. Government intervention means that the health-care burden is evenly spread. The tax, of course, is high.

The choice—government subsidizing both the rich and the poor or subsidizing only the poor—is a political one. We pay through taxes, or we pay through savings. If you think only of taxes, it is cheaper to subsidize just the poor. But if we then were to become miserly and did not provide enough aid, poor and chronically ill patients, and those with expensive illnesses, will suffer disproportionately. But luck will be the major determinant of your family's finances. Luck will dictate whether you can or cannot afford medical care. The purpose of government intervention is to reduce the effect of luck on your fate. The world's richest nation should not permit chance illness to take families down.

Rationing means less care. How much *less* can we give and still be humane? What are the boundaries of *care*? Does it include medications, eyeglasses, and treatment for a common cold? Physical therapy for the moribund? Does it include home health care, drug treatment clinics, and nutritious school lunches? Before we consider rationing, we must formally address these questions and answer them unambiguously.

Should we treat only treatable disease? Society benefits little in a financial sense when a terminal cancer is palliated, an advanced AIDS patient is hospitalized, a stroke patient is rehabilitated, or a kidney-failure patient is put on a dialysis machine. But we still do these things. If cost-benefit were our only criterion for care we might not. In a cost-benefit system, regardless who suffers, a minor illness which gets better on its own is not reimbursed, nor is a major illness for which there is no effective cure. Thus some of the patients who cannot pay out of pocket are ineligible for treatment. This form of exclusion discriminates by luck of diagnosis. You can justify it by saying that nature, not man, has been unfair—if that salves your conscience at all.

The trick of doing cost-benefit rationing wisely is to include quality of life in the equation, and not to ignore the cost of alternative care, to understand that years of a nursing home may cost more than a hip replacement. It seems simple in principle. However, to understand *all* the costs, to anticipate *all* the benefits may make cost-benefit rationing too complex to apply.

Cost-benefit alone cannot be the single criterion for care. Human compassion must be a guideline as well. Besides, in treating the "incurable" we doctors learn how to cure. Within our memory, tuberculosis was a lethal disease. Heart attacks were once death sentences, and the average survival of a lupus patient was three years. Lessons learned by treating the untreatable have enabled us eventually to devise cures. Most cost-benefit analyses think only in the short term. We must also consider the long-term gain of treating "incurable" disease.

Is there a minimum quality of life below which, or a maximum age beyond which patients should not expect medical care? A yes answer to either question diminishes the value of the lives of those who cannot speak for themselves. Coma is the state that most often spurs this discussion, but idiocy, dementia, severe genetic and congenital disease, even mental illness are quickly mentioned. There is no footnote to the Declaration of Geneva that adds "except when (in the doctor's judgment) life is not worth living." I can withdraw medical care on a patient's request, but I cannot do so on your request when the patient says No.

In our society we do not—yet—exclude on the basis of age or membership in a particular group. The potential for abuse of such a criterion is immense. You see the problem more clearly if you think about other exclusion criteria you might use. Substitute the word "black" or "woman" for "aged," and see how the concept sounds. Let your imagination soar. Exclude the ugly, the unintelligent, the redheads. Does this exclusion sound reprehensible? If so, then exclusion because of age does, too.

Should those who abuse their bodies share in the cost of repair? This question has merit, is even attractive if you think only of drug abuse or violence. But as I have suggested, to start formulating acceptable and unacceptable definitions of self-abuse is to start on a very slippery slope. To most people, heroin addiction is bad. To others, a beef and dairy diet is, too. To still others, skiing and hockey should be outlawed. We have no clear definitions of self-abuse, or of exemplary self-care.

Should we ration medical care by self-selection? We can formally distinguish between health maintenance and illness care. We could give everyone a level of minimum health maintenance care and care in dealing with minor illnesses, then offer voluntary insurance to cover the costs of expensive chronic diseases. This would be self-selection—people who buy the insurance will receive all the care they request, and those who don't will get only the minimum. But this form of rationing can and would harm the unwise or the uninformed. Furthermore, it is very difficult for poor people to order priorities—to pay for housing *or* food *or* health care. A democracy is supposed to protect its weakest members. Self-selected rationing does not fulfill this goal.

Should we ration medical care through the marketplace? We already do. One in seven of us is uninsured—and that's a form of rationing. In marketplace rationing, financial gatekeepers decide, according to inconsistent rules, what care patients will receive. The uninsured and the unemployed are excluded. Marketplace rationing abandons the person who does not or cannot provide for himself. It discriminates against those with chronic illness and against those who cannot speak for themselves. With no city hospitals, no safety nets, and no treatment at all, marketplace rationing mocks our nation's best values.

Should we ration medical care by centrally limiting resources? Once, long ago, I had a conversation about how to share twenty respirators (iron lungs) among the more than twenty patients then on a pulmonary ward. One doctor said that a decision would be easy in his native Delhi: that city, it seemed, had but one respirator—a rationed resource; with only one respirator, it was inexpensive to care for patients with severe lung disease because they quickly died. In the United States today, Delhi's respirator might be an organ transplantation, or gene transfer, or dialysis, even a coronary bypass. In the United States as in Delhi, death is cheaper than chronic care.

If we ration technology, wealthy patients could still purchase it from private vendors. If we cannot afford to provide all care to all people, if we agree to provide a minimum level of service for everyone and at some central point limit the available resources, we have made a moral, but agonizing, choice. The rich will suffer less, of course. They always do.

What priority does health care have in our total public budget? In theory, it ought to be simple to set a budget priority. Decide first the value of the item, and how much we can afford, then determine a compromise number. We can do this exercise for all the federal budget items—defense, education, infrastructure, energy. Put them all together and compromise again, and there you have it, the priorities have been established. It ought to be simple, if all the needs have been specified and if we have put all the items simultaneously on the table.

It might be that we would give health care a high priority, even that we would choose to pay for maximum health care for all citizens. It may be that we will vote to palliate the incurable and to sustain the disabled. It may be that we will support the use of the most advanced services regardless of an individual patient's ability to pay. It may be that we will wish our government, not private corporations, to broker this choice.

If so, health care will cost a much higher proportion of our national wealth. To afford it, we can either pay higher taxes or apportion our taxes differently. In a peaceful world there may be no defense costs: we could reduce that portion of our national budget and add the saving to health care. If we reduce our exorbitant national consumption, the cost of maintaining our infrastructure would fall. If the world becomes more just, public safety expenses might be less. There is no magic amount that we need to spend or not spend for health care.

We do need to decide.

We can save wasted money, negotiate fees, and ration services. To make a big difference, we have to reassess the very basis of what we are doing. We must ask what the goals of medical care are, what the boundaries of care are, and whether we should support it with public or private funds. We must establish a priority for health care's share of those funds. We must make these decisions coherently, and we must answer each question with a clear yes or with a clear no.

So we come full circle. We must complete the schoolbook exercise in the last chapter. We must face the questions head-on. How would *you* save money? What do *you* want from medical care? What is the limit of *your* charity?

If you have good answers, speak them aloud. Tell your representative and senator. Tell your newspaper. Tell me.

CONCLUSION: GUARDED PROGNOSIS

The United States has an outstanding health-care system. We have the best doctors, the best hospitals, and the best medical research that have ever been. This health-care system is costly, and to reduce the cost, we are now reshaping the system. But there have been no pilot studies and no experimentation. Analysis has been incomplete.

To dabble unthoughtfully, to attack the current most visible and urgent problem and not to see it as part of the whole, will unbalance the health-care entropy. Doctors know from experience with patients (amateur auto mechanics know this principle, too) that catastrophes follow careless tinkering. A solution that alters one component—for instance, the dollars devoted to medical care for our elderly population—irrevocably alters another. Reduce the number of hip replacements and you increase the number of disabled people. Raise the age of Medicare eligibility and you increase unemployment, because older workers will not retire as soon as they do now. Push the balloon here, and it bulges there.

I have no certainty that what is now happening will harm us. Possibly the prognosis for a less expensive health-care system is very good. But it is also possible that the new changes will cause irremediable harm. It is possible, even probable, that the prognosis for our health-care system is guarded—meaning very poor. As we enter the unknown, I dislike what I see happening to individual patients, to vulnerable people with chronic diseases and to people who are of advanced age.

The changes have already begun. Some parts of the old fee-for-service illness care were good and should be retained. Some parts of the new health maintenance are also good. Ideally, we should borrow what is good from both the old and the new and discard that which no longer serves.

An ideal system must have these elements:

- Universal access to medical care, in a system in which the patient as well as the provider has a say in what happens.
- Both health maintenance and illness care, which guarantee that very ill patients will not be cast aside.
- Portability of health insurance, not only between jobs but in different geographic areas, including guarantees that people will not lose their doctors when their employer selects a new plan.
- Detaching physicians' income from the individual services they provide, so that they do not become adversaries of their patients.
- Rationing on a national or at least a regional level, not a local one, so that a few patients do not determine the many's access to medical care.

- Continuity, especially for patients with chronic disease.
- Reduction of the administrative burdens.

The stories in this book illustrate the problems that need solutions. On the surface, the problems seem medical, but they are social and political as well. The stories ask: When the aggregate costs are the main concern, how can we be sure we are protecting individuals? And when our policies are modeled on the idea of simple, short-term illness, are they harmful to those who have complex and chronic disease?

It is possible to address these questions with more humanity than we have yet done. In public debates, we now ask questions mostly about aggregate populations—how much we should pay for old people's care, for example. The answers are objective and very abstract. If you ask the same questions about individuals, the answers are poignant and more concrete. Abstract policies affect individual people, and we must keep them in mind. It is still possible to protect each person. It is still possible to be humane.

Before Medicare and Medicaid, the "system" did not work well for Fred Thomas. A decade later, Tia Hendricks controlled her own medical care. In an era of conventional health insurance, no one questioned the efforts that allowed Alice Tsang and Brenda O'Neill to survive. We once said: Of course, the Weintraubs and the Rubins can have a child, and did not ask how much it would cost.

We are wiser now. We know the price for all these decisions. As a result, formal rationing of health care is very likely to occur. Who—patients, doctors, government, or industry—will decide what to ration? Who will set the limits on individual medical care?

Those who are most affected—those who suffer from chronic illness, those who are disabled, and those who are poor—must speak their minds. Their voices are not loud, so others must join them. Do they, or do you, have the information that you need?

We have not had much informed public debate on these matters. We are now embracing a new system of health care whose implications we have not thought through. So let us now debate, openly, boisterously, the futures of *both* health maintenance *and* illness care. Let us consider the options and construct our medical systems accordingly. Let us not forget that individual people, very vulnerable ones, feel the blows of or are protected by every "Yes" and "No." We should have public debate on how to limit medical costs, so long as that debate considers *individual* need. Those who are ill must speak for themselves. Their voices are not being heard in the present cacophony. In repeating their stories, we add our voices to theirs.

Before you cast your ballot in this debate, put before your eyes the face and voice of just one person who might be affected by your vote. Imagine yourself face to face with her—she is asking for help, and you alone are deciding whether to pay for her care. And please do not imagine that you can decide against her and have someone else execute the command. You alone will tell that person your decision—as I, a doctor, now have to tell my patients what I am or am not permitted to do. Will you be able to say, "In your case, I have said No"? If it were your mother, your father, your spouse, or your child, or any of the persons in these pages, would your answer still be No?

Please do not ask your doctor to tell a patient about a choice that is in fact yours. When commercial goals and the interests of the individual patient diverge, do not ask your doctor to *pretend* to support his patient but in truth to support the corporation.

That is not what doctors do.

It is not what this doctor will do.

EPILOGUE

Missing patients, I returned to patients.

Missing New York, I came back to New York.

My former patients and colleagues greeted me ardently, women hugging, men shaking hands. This type of greeting is pleasant but not a surprise. Hugs and handshakes are, after all, the currency of American discourse. Yet some of the greetings were a bit disconcerting: One patient of mine ran up and hugged me as I was speaking to a full conference room. I enjoyed the greetings, but a new perspective gave me the most pleasure.

Invited to two *bar mitzvahs* of my patients' children, uncertain of the dates when I would return to town, I had given only tentative yes's in my RSVPs. But I was in town and I did attend. At the first ceremony I chose a seat near the back, not wanting my presence to remind the boy's family of past illness and thus detract from the joy of the day.

I needn't have been so self-conscious. Most *bar mitzvah*

speeches are predictable, but this one startled me. Perhaps startled is an inadequate word: the French *bouleversé* is better. "I first appeared in print," the boy began, "in the *New England Journal of Medicine* in the spring of 1985." Now *that* was an original opening line. In those seventeen words he introduced to the congregation the medical paper in which I had described clinical details of his very frightening birth. He went on to speak about what his mother had endured and about the high chance that he might have died; he described his mother's current good health. He said he felt special to have grown to manhood with a rare knowledge.

Two weeks later a girl who neither knew the boy nor had heard what he said, at her *bat mitzvah* also spoke of her tenuous first days and of her mother's illness. She talked about kidney failure, dialysis, and transplantation—from a daughter's point of view—and at the end of her speech she handed out organ donation cards.

For both speeches, the entire congregations were in tears. The sight of this boy and this girl, thriving and confident, of their healthy mothers, says more forcefully by example than I can: we must make available the medical choices we made thirteen years ago to patients today. It *is* important that we do all that we can for those who suffer from chronic and catastrophic disease.

On my first day back in New York, a colleague took me to the bedside of Keisha Franklin's sister, now very ill. Nauseated, somnolent, confused, she looked at me, puzzled, when I entered her room. Then she blinked, shook her head, stared for a minute or two, and said my name. Another hug.

Christina Papadopoulos did not try to become pregnant again. She has a new kidney; Raizl Weintraub is waiting for one.

Winnie Brown recently had a small stroke. Her twelve-year-old son gave his mother emergency care, called the ambulance, and located his father (a motorman for the New York subways!) at work. She recovered, but not fully, and can no longer hold a job.

Before Dr. Saeeda Hasan died, her daughter married and her son entered college; she was very pleased.

Sandra Richards is more or less well. Her daughter Ruth is very bright.

After fifteen months, Melissa Poggi began to speak, but eight years later, she can still say only a few words. She cannot control her arms or legs, feed, or bathe herself. The cost of her care remains high.

Brenda O'Neill is well. So were Ella Redgrave and Susan Sandman the last I heard.

Hubert Steiner still uses canes to walk. He has invented many devices that help him overcome the disabilities that he still has.

I have lost contact with Gloria Bermudez, Jean-Paul Pelletier, Hélène Duval, Peter Malone, and Mavis Green.

Other patients, with new problems, have taken the places of those who are gone. There will be more patients still to come. In the near future my patients and I will make decisions together. I hope these decisions will be made by us alone, or by my patients with my advice. I hope their life decisions will not be made for them by strangers.

INDEX